UNDERSTANDING WATER, EI
AND ACID-BASE BALANCE

CW01017916

Understanding Water, Electrolyte and Acid-base Balance

PETER RICHARDS, MA MD PhD FRCP

Professor of Medicine and Dean
St Mary's Hospital Medical School
University of London

and

BRUNO TRUNIGER, Dr Med

Professor of Medicine
Chefarzt Medizinische Klinik
Kantonsspital Luzern
Switzerland

WILLIAM HEINEMANN MEDICAL BOOKS LTD

London

First published 1983

© Peter Richards and Bruno Truniger, 1983

ISBN 0-433-27593-6

Printed in Great Britain at The Pitman Press, Bath

'yf I have sayed a misse, I am content that any man amende it, or yf I have sayd to lytle, any man that wyl to add what hym pleaseth to it.'

'My mind is . . . that youthe myght by styrred to labour, honest pastyme, and vertue . . .'

Roger Ascham
Toxophilus, the Schole of Shootinge
London, 1545

Contents

Preface

A practical understanding of the role of body fluids in the pathogenesis and treatment of disease brings great benefits to patients at little cost.

This book should be read for the first time during the introduction to clinical medicine and surgery, reserving the Appendix for later. It should then be read in its entirety a few months before the qualifying examinations. Finally, the Appendix should be used to provide a framework for sensible action in individual problems during the early days of clinical practice.

Our approach to fluid and electrolyte disturbances builds on, but does not repeat, the basic renal and endocrine physiology taught in the early years of the medical course. We have concentrated on information which we have found clinically useful ourselves and we have tried to give a perspective in the Tables by underlining the most common conditions. Although the principles apply to children, the relative importance of different conditions in childhood and the details of their treatment are outside the scope of this book.

We warmly thank Sir Douglas Black, Professor Hugh Dudley and Professor John Owen, physician, surgeon and chemical pathologist respectively, for generously giving their constructive criticisms and Dr David Brooks for helping us to cut the final version to size. Any remaining errors and imperfections are entirely ours.

Peter Richards   Bruno Truniger
London   Luzern

June, 1983

1.

The Boundaries of Disturbance

Electrolytes are salts, acids and bases which dissociate in aqueous solution into electrically-charged particles. In the dilute solution found in body fluids some electrolytes dissociate almost completely (such as neutral salts, e.g. sodium chloride) and others dissociate to only a small extent (such as organic acids and bases, e.g. carbonic acid).

Electrolytes contribute to health and disease both by their entirely non-specific osmotic properties as particles in solution and by their own specific ionic properties.

THE OSMOLALITY OF BODY FLUIDS

Osmotic pressure is the pressure which must be applied to the solution at one side of a membrane which is permeable to solvent but not to solute molecules in order to prevent solvent from entering the solution. Cell membranes act as a semipermeable membrane in this respect: they are impermeable to the polyvalent anions within them and are in effect impermeable to sodium outside them because the sodium-pump mechanism actively extrudes sodium from the cell; they are freely permeable to water.

Because cell membranes are freely permeable to water extracellular fluid (ECF) and intracellular fluid (ICF) are isotonic i.e. they have the same osmolality (*see below*). The osmolality of ECF is regulated by means of the hypothalamic 'osmostat' (p. 24) which normally maintains a constant plasma osmolality because a 1% rise in plasma osmolality triggers both thirst and the release of antidiuretic hormone (ADH) with the result that more water is both taken in and retained; a fall in plasma osmolality has the opposite effects. An increase in plasma (and ECF) osmolality also

1

results in an osmotic water movement from ICF and ECF; a fall in plasma osmolality has the opposite effect.

The osmolality of a solution is a reflection of the number of osmotically active particles within it; it is routinely measured rapidly and simply by measuring vapour pressure or depression of freezing point and expressed per kg of water either as mmol (SI units) or mosmol. One osmole of a substance depresses the freezing point of water by $1.86\,°C$; one milliosmole is one thousandth of an osmole.

The osmolality of a solution containing a number of solutes is close to (but slightly less than) the sum of their individual osmolalities: for example, 1 mole of sodium chloride dissociates into 1 mole of sodium ions and 1 mole of chloride ions, i.e. two osmotically active particles giving an osmolality twice the molality if completely dissociated and in a very dilute solution; a compound formed from a divalent cation and univalent anion, such as sodium sulphate (Na_2SO_4) would have an osmolality three times the molality under the same conditions. Most of the osmotically important constituents of plasma are univalent electrolytes, sodium chloride predominating. The plasma osmolality attributable to electrolytes can be calculated approximately (provided plasma proteins and lipids are not substantially increased) as follows:

$$\frac{\text{Plasma osmolality}}{\text{(mmol/kg water)}} = \frac{\text{Plasma sodium}}{\text{(mmol/l)} \times 2}$$

This relationship holds by a chance cancelling out of two factors. Plasma is approximately 6.5% solids (mainly protein) so that the concentration of plasma electrolytes per litre has to be multiplied by 1.07 to express them per kg of plasma water. The factor by which the concentration has to be diminished to take account of the osmotic coefficient is by chance almost identical (*see* Table 1.1).

Plasma osmolality, therefore, normally closely reflects the plasma sodium concentration. As plasma osmolality is kept constant, it follows that the amount of sodium in ECF determines the volume of ECF. It also follows that the total body water will be determined largely by the total exchangeable

Table 1.1
CALCULATED OSMOLALITY OF AVERAGE NORMAL
PLASMA

Component	Concentration mmol/l	Molality mmol/kg of water	Osmotic‡ coefficient	Osmolality mmol/kg of water
Sodium	140	148	0.94	140
Chloride	100	106	0.92	98
Bicarbonate	23	24	0.75	18
Other electrolytes	7*	7	0.90†	6
Glucose	5	5	1.01	5
Urea	3	3	0.99	3
Other non-electrolytes	15*	16	1.00	16
				286

* Estimated
† Assumed value
‡ The ratio of the osmolality of the solute to its molality at body temperature and at plasma concentration (From Owen J.A., Edwards R.G., Coller B.A.W. (1970). *The Mole in Medicine and Biology*, p. 39. Edinburgh: Livingstone.)

sodium and potassium in the body (potassium being the major intracellular cation).

If ECF osmolality rises, water moves from ICF to ECF; a fall in ECF osmolality causes movement in the opposite direction. The distribution of ECF between interstitial and vascular spaces depends primarily on the plasma colloid osmotic pressure ('oncotic' pressure) (*see* p. 13), which is largely determined by the plasma albumin concentration.

The normal plasma osmolality is 290–300 mmol/kg of water. The deviations which can be tolerated depend largely upon the speed at which they develop. If the disturbance develops slowly, a plasma osmolality as low as 230 or as high as 360 mmol/kg can be tolerated with few symptoms. But profound symptoms ensue with a much smaller deviation if the disturbance is rapid.

Table 1.2
THE COMPOSITION AND OSMOLALITY OF COMMONLY USED INTRAVENOUS SOLUTIONS OF WATER AND ELECTROLYTES

Solution	Glucose mmol/l	Na mmol/l	K mmol/l	Cl mmol/l	HCO_3 or equiv mmol/l	Calcium mmol/l	Theoretical osmolality* mmol/kg
Dextrose (5%)	278	—	—	—	—	—	278
Sodium chloride (0.9%) ('Normal saline')	—	150	—	150	—	—	300
Sodium chloride (0.18%) & Dextrose (4.3%)	239	30	—	30	—	—	299
Sodium bicarbonate (1.4%) (M/6)	—	167	—	—	167	—	334
Sodium lactate (1.9%) (M/6)	—	167	—	—	167	—	334
Compound sodium lactate (Hartmann's solution)	—	131	5	111	27 (as lactate)	2	276
Sodium bicarbonate (8.4%) (used in cardiac arrest)	—	1000	—	—	1000	—	2000

* The effective osmolality is slightly less (*see* osmolal coefficient Table 1.1)

Table 1.3
COMMON ELECTROLYTES IN GRAM/MOLAR UNITS

Sodium chloride	1	mmol	58.5	mg
	17	mmol	1	g
Sodium bicarbonate	1	mmol	84	mg
	11.9	mmol	1	g
Potassium chloride	1	mmol	74.5	mg
	13.4	mmol	1	g
Calcium gluconate	1	mmol	448	mg
(hydrated)	2.2	mmol	1	g*
Magnesium chloride	1	mmol	204	mg
(hydrated)	4.9	mmol	1	g

* Contains 90 mg of calcium

The terms 'isotonic', 'physiological' or 'normal' in relation to body fluids take as their reference point the normal osmolality of plasma. The osmolality of the most commonly used intravenous electrolyte solutions are given in Table 1.2. The mg/mmol relationships of the physiologically most important electrolytes are given in Table 1.3.

DISTRIBUTION OF SODIUM, POTASSIUM AND WATER

Intracellular Fluid (ICF) and Extracellular Fluid (ECF)

The chemical composition of ECF (in which Na and Cl predominate) is radically different from ICF (in which K and PO_4 predominate) partly because of the intracellular anions (mainly protein and organic phosphate) to which cell membranes are impermeable and partly because of the Na-pump mechanism which actively expels Na from cells in exchange for K.

It is worth repeating that the only common feature of ECF and ICF is their osmolality. Most cell membranes are freely permeable to water and administered water distributes rapidly throughout ICF and ECF (excluding bone, cartilage and dense connective tissue), which together with a small amount of transcellular fluid comprise the total body water (TBW). TBW accounts for 50–70% of body weight in adults (*see* p. 24).

Readily exchangeable water in ICF is twice the volume of

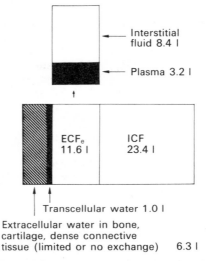

Fig 1.1 Distribution of body water in a 70 kg patient. ECF_e = readily exchangeable extracellular fluid. *Note*: the 2:1 (23.4:11.551) ratio of $ICF:ECF_e$ differs from the traditional physiological teaching which offers a ratio of 55:45% or 23.4:18.91 to include in the ECF 6.31 of fluid in bone, cartilage and dense connective tissue, as well as 1.051 of transcellular fluid (glandular secretions) not normally relevant in clinical calculations. (From Edelman I.S., Leibman J. (1959). Anatomy of body water and electrolytes. *Amer. J. Med*; 27:256–77.)

ECF, the approximate values being given in Fig 1.1. ECF is comprised of plasma and interstitial fluid in the proportions shown in Fig 1.1. A small proportion of total body water is transcellular, sequestered in secretions of which the largest component is fluid within the gastrointestinal tract.

Figure 1.2 summarises the major differences in the composition of ICF and ECF. Intracellular values are difficult to determine accurately and the composition of intracellular fluid of different tissues varies: the figures in Fig 1.2 are derived from skeletal muscle.

The active extrusion of sodium from cells sets up a membrane potential with the inside negatively charged in relation to the outside surface. This negative potential within cells repels the entry of negatively-charged anions, such as chloride, and favours the accumulation of potassium. A dynamic steady-state is created in which electroneutrality and osmotic balance are achieved.

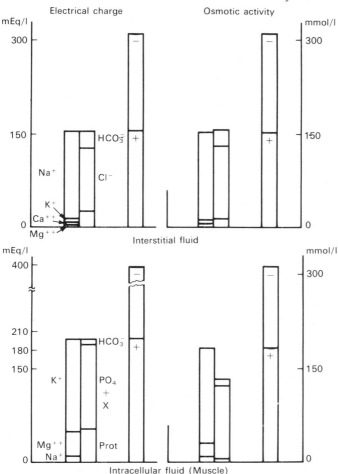

Fig 1.2 The electroneutrality and osmolar equality of ECF (blood plasma and interstitial fluid) and ICF. *Note*: the electrical charges of cations and anions must balance in ECF and ICF. The concentrations of osmotically active particles must be the same in ECF and ICF. There are slightly more divalent cations in ECF than anions and the number of cationic particles is, therefore, slightly smaller than the number of anionic particles. In ICF the difference is reversed and substantially greater, the polyvalent intracellular anions being a large molecular size but lesser in number. The sum of osmotically active particles is, however, the same in ECF and ICF whatever the difference in terms of anions and cations. X = other organic anions. (Adapted from Gamble J.L. (1954). *Chemical Anatomy, Physiology and Pathology of Extracellular Fluid*. Cambridge, Mass: Harvard University Press.)

If, however, the supply of metabolic energy is diminished, the sodium pump falters, sodium accumulates in cells and chloride ions enter to balance the charges; less potassium enters the cell in coupled exchange for sodium, potassium is no longer retained to the same extent within cells and is more easily able to leave the cell down the concentration gradient. The net result of these changes is an increase in intracellular solute (sodium and chloride ingress exceeding potassium loss), water moves in to preserve isotonicity between ECF and ICF and the cell swells. When sufficient metabolic energy is re-provided the processes are reversed and cell size returns to normal. About one-third of the resting energy requirement of cells is used to maintain constant cell volume.

Effects of Water and Saline Loads and Losses upon the Composition of ICF and ECF

A water load distributes rapidly throughout the body fluids; ICF and ECF are expanded in proportion to their initial volume. An isotonic dextrose solution (278 mmol/l; 5 g%) is used as a convenient way of infusing water without electrolyte and avoiding the danger of lysing red cells. The infused water distributes throughout total body water just as rapidly as the glucose is metabolised or enters cells. Diagrammatically this situation can be represented as in Fig. 1.3: in a 70 kg man 3 l of 5% dextrose expand the ICF by 2 l and ECF by 1 l if none of the water is excreted (A);

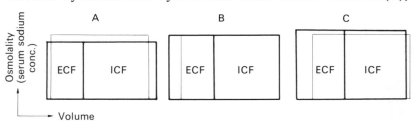

Fig 1.3 Changes in volume and concentration (osmolality) of ICF and ECF on administration of equal amounts of water (as 5% dextrose) (A), isotonic saline (B), and hypertonic saline (C). Compartments enclosed by thin lines represent the initial normal state; those enclosed by heavy lines represent the final experimental state. Modified and reproduced with permission from Pitts R.F.: *Physiology of the Kidney and Body Fluids*, 3rd edn. Copyright © 1974 by Year Book Medical Publishers, Inc., Chicago. (Adapted from Darrow D.C. and Yannet H.: *Clin. Invest.*; **14**:266, 1935.)

plasma water comprises one-quarter of the readily exchangeable ECF and therefore increases only by about 150 ml. In contrast, infusion of 3 l of isotonic saline expands only the ECF (B). The increase is about 25% (3 l in 11.55 l) and plasma volume is increased in proportion by 800 ml, an amount sufficient to precipitate heart failure in a patient with poor cardiac function.

Administration of hypertonic saline expands the ECF at the expense of ICF water because water moves from ICF to ECF until the osmolality is again equal in ECF and ICF. The final osmolality in both compartments is increased at equilibrium (C). Administration of 1 l of 2 N saline (twice 'normal' *see* p. 5) expands the ECF to almost the same extent as 2 l of N saline, because the additional water is extracted from ICF. Repeated administration of hypertonic saline is therefore potentially dangerous both because of ECF overload and ICF contraction.

The converse of these situations holds. Water losses are sustained by ECF and ICF in simple proportion to their initial volume. Loss of sodium and water in fluid hypotonic to plasma (e.g. sweat) depletes both ECF and ICF but the loss from ECF is proportionately greater than if the loss had been of water alone. Isotonic saline loss reduces only ECF volume and does not alter plasma osmolality.

A net deficit of sodium chloride in excess of water relative to the normal composition of plasma develops when salt and water deficit is corrected with water alone and, rarely, in sodium-losing renal disease (when sodium loss is proportionately greater than water loss): the net effect is equivalent to loss of hypertonic saline (although no body fluids except occasionally urine contain sodium chloride in higher concentration than plasma); ECF volume and osmolality are reduced as a direct result of the saline loss and ECF volume is further reduced by an osmotic movement of water from the now hypotonic ECF to ICF to equalise their osmolality.

Clinical Recognition of Deficit and Excess of Water and of Saline

Confusion arising from use of the term 'dehydration'

Although 'dehydration' literally means water depletion, the term is used with wider meaning in clinical practice to describe the signs and symptoms produced by reduced ECF volume i.e. the effects of salt and water depletion. Pure water deficiency is less common than a combined deficiency of salt and water, and pure water depletion has to be very severe before ECF volume is diminished to a clinically apparent extent (because the water deficit is distributed throughout total body water, ICF + ECF, while saline depletion predominantly reduces the much smaller ECF volume). Clinical licence in the use of the term dehydration is so universal as to be beyond correction, but the importance of being clear that the term is generally used to mean ECF deficit due to both water *and* salt deficiency cannot be too strongly emphasised.

Water depletion (ICF and ECF depletion)

Water deficit is distributed over total body water (42 l in a 70 kg man); a 4 l water deficit therefore only reduces both ICF and ECF by 10%, a deficit which causes thirst (by increasing plasma osmolality) but no signs until plasma volume suffers, by which stage the overall deficit is likely to be about 8 l and the patient almost dead. The urine volume is small and the urine is highly concentrated (> 700 mmol/kg) provided renal function and control of ADH is normal. Plasma sodium and albumin concentrations are increased and so is the haemoglobin concentration. In short, a much larger pure water loss is tolerated without signs of ECF depletion than is possible with saline loss. The major symptoms and signs of water deficiency are summarised in Table 1.4.

Water excess (ECF and ICF expansion)

Water excess is not tolerated as well as deficit because water excess causes cell swelling and the extent to which the brain can swell without a symptomatic rise in intracranial pressure is small. Confusion is usually the first symptom (*see* Table 1.4). The plasma sodium, albumin and the haemoglobin are all low, reflecting haemodilution. The urine is very dilute provided ADH secretion is suppressed normally; frequently, however, failure to suppress ADH secretion is the cause of water intoxication.

Although the plasma sodium concentration is low, urinary

Table 1.4
MAJOR SYMPTOMS AND SIGNS OF PURE WATER (TBW)
DEPLETION AND EXCESS

A. *Depletion*
1. Thirst, confusion and other neurological signs in severe cases
2. Urine highly concentrated (>700 mmol/kg) if renal function and control of ADH release normal
3. Plasma osmolality raised: hypernatraemia
4. Raised haemoglobin (provided no anaemia)
5. Plasma albumin raised (provided no other disease)
6. Loss of weight

B. *Excess*
1. Confusion (and later other neurological signs of cerebral oedema: eventually coma)
2. Urine very dilute (if renal function and ADH control normal and no ectopic source of ADH) – to a minimum of 70 mmol/kg
3. Plasma osmolality reduced: hyponatraemia
4. Low haemoglobin
5. Low plasma albumin
6. Increase in weight

sodium excretion is not reduced, in fact it increases in response to the expanded circulatory volume (*see* p. 30).

Saline depletion (ECF deficit)

Reduced ECF volume becomes clinically apparent largely through the effects of reduced plasma volume, but also through reduction in interstitial fluid. The major symptoms and signs are listed in Table 1.5. Thirst is a late symptom if plasma osmolality is unchanged, becoming apparent only when plasma volume is reduced sufficiently to cause hypotension. In this situation thirst is probably mediated by angiotensin release.

Saline excess (ECF expansion)

The symptoms and signs of saline excess are summarised in Table 1.5. The first sign is an increase in body weight; the jugular venous pressure rises (unless the plasma albumin concentration is low) and oedema develops when ECF has increased by about 5 l in an average adult.

Table 1.5
MAJOR SYMPTOMS AND SIGNS OF SALINE (ECF)
DEPLETION AND EXCESS

A. *Depletion*
1. General weakness
2. Thirst (a late symptom – *see text*)
3. Cardiovascular
    Exaggereated postural fall in blood pressure
    Jugular venous filling not visible at 45° and sometimes not when
        lying flat
    Peripheral vasoconstriction (a late sign)
    Complete absence of pulmonary crepitations
    CXR: reduced heart size (if old films available for comparison)
4. Urine (provided renal function is normal)
    Small volume
    Usually, but not invariably highly concentrated
        (>700 mmol/kg of water)
    Low sodium concentration (<20 mmol/l)

Note. We do not find the following traditional signs to be useful in
practice in adults:
    reduced tissue turgor (difficult to differentiate from wasting)
    dry mouth (because many ill patients mouth-breathe)
    reduced intraocular pressure (a very late sign)

B. *Excess*
1. Recent increase in weight
2. Cardiovascular
    Dyspnoea ± orthopnoea
    Oedema (peripheral, sacral and possibly pulmonary)
    Jugular venous pressure raised (unless plasma albumin concentra-
        tion low)
    Pulmonary crepitations
    CXR: cardiac enlargement; pulmonary venous congestion,
        pleural effusions ± septal oedema
3. Urine
    Findings dependent on the cause of overload (*see* Table 3.1)

The mechanisms of peripheral oedema are well explained in
principle by the Starling hypothesis (Fig 1.4).

   1. The force favouring escape of plasma water with its
      diffusible solutes at the arteriolar end of capillaries is:
      arteriolar capillary hydrostatic pressure.

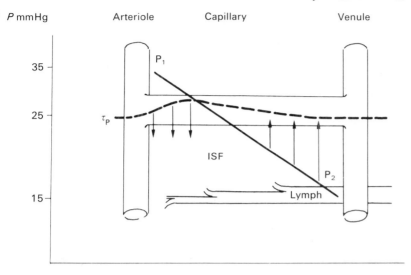

Fig 1.4 Forces acting upon the movement of fluid from capillaries to interstitial space and *vice versa* (Starling forces). P_1 and P_2 refer to the intracapillary (hydrostatic) pressure at the arteriolar (P_1) and the venular (P_2) end of the capillary. τ_p is the colloid osmotic pressure of the plasma as modified by filtration and reabsorption of protein free fluid. The difference between hydrostatic and oncotic pressures in and outside the capillary normally favour filtration at the arteriolar, reabsorption at the venular end of the capillary. (From Boylan J. W., Deetjen P., Kramer K. (1970). Niere und Wasserhausalt. Vol III. In *Physiologie des Menschen* (Gauer O.H., Kramer K., Jung R. eds) Munchen: Urban and Schwarzenberg.

2. The forces limiting its escape from the arteriolar capillary
   and favouring its return at the venous end of capillaries are:
      oncotic pressure of plasma proteins (*see* p. 3)
      tissue elasticity, resisting distension ('tissue turgor').
3. The forces limiting the return of interstitial fluid to capillaries are:
      venous capillary hydrostatic pressure (which is increased
      in heart failure or if there is local venous obstruction)
      the normally small oncotic pressure of interstitial fluid.
4. Interstitial fluid is continuously being drained into
   lymphatics; lymphatic blockage predisposes to oedema
   (lymphoedema).

The Central Venous Pressure (CVP) as a Guide to Fluid Balance and Therapy

The height of the jugular venous pressure is a useful indicator of plasma volume and of the presence or absence of right heart failure. Precise measurement of the central venous pressure by a central venous catheter is particularly useful in guiding the volume of fluid replacement in acute illness. Care must be taken to avoid any technical pitfalls such as blocked or malpositioned catheters and to interpret measurements in the context of the whole clinical picture.

Central venous pressure gives an indication of both right ventricular function and of postcapillary plasma volume; both impairment of right ventricular function and expansion of plasma volume raise the CVP and ECF deficiency results in a fall. This does not, however, necessarily mean that replacement of plasma volume can be planned against the CVP measurement alone because left ventricular failure (which is insensitively monitored by the CVP) may in various circumstances precede the full correction of plasma volume deficiency; this applies both to replacement of blood and to correction of ECF deficiency with saline.

It is important to appreciate that salt and water replacement in a dehydrated patient cannot easily be judged from the CVP if the plasma albumin concentration is low; plasma volume is low because plasma oncotic pressure is reduced and plasma volume cannot be restored to normal by infusion of sodium and water without, at the same time, causing peripheral and pulmonary oedema.

The CVP is an insensitive marker of absolute water excess or deficiency because plasma volume is affected only in the same proportion as all body fluids.

THE SIGNIFICANCE OF THE PLASMA SODIUM CONCENTRATION

A raised plasma sodium concentration always signifies increased plasma osmolality. A low plasma sodium concentration does not necessarily indicate reduced osmolality because other osmotically active plasma constituents, such as glucose, may be simultaneously increased. Also, if plasma water is reduced on account of an increased concentration of lipoproteins or gammaglobulins, the sodium concentration measured per litre of plasma will be reduced although its concentration per litre of plasma water (and therefore the osmolality of plasma is unchanged; a spuriously low plasma sodium concentration in this situation is sometimes referred to as 'pseudohyponatraemia'.

Plasma sodium concentration by itself gives no information concerning the total amount of either sodium or water in the body. Both the plasma sodium and plasma osmolality simply reflect the *relative* amounts of sodium and water; hyponatraemia (and a low plasma osmolality) indicates relative water excess; hypernatraemia (and a raised plasma osmolality) indicates relative water deficiency; a normal plasma sodium indicates normal relative proportions. Figure 1.5 illustrates the impossibility of drawing conclusions about absolute amounts of sodium and water from their relative proportions in plasma.

Clinical assessment of evidence for fluid depletion or excess (Tables 1.4; 1.5) is fundamental to the interpretation of plasma sodium concentration and osmolality. For example, if a hyponatraemic patient shows signs of saline depletion and the urine sodium concentration is low (<10 mmol/l), indicating a normal renal response to sodium deficiency, the patient is suffering either from salt and water loss by a non-renal route, i.e. from gastrointestinal loss or from increased sweating, or from severe restriction of intake. Alternatively the patient may recently have been taking a diuretic but now have stopped. A higher urinary sodium concentration in these circumstances indicates failure of normal renal conservation as a result of either renal or adrenal disease. In all these circumstances the low plasma sodium concentration indicates that sodium loss or restriction has been proportionately greater than that of water.

If a hyponatraemic patient is oedematous, he is suffering from salt and water overload (because the oedema fluid is ECF and ECF is saline) but the water overload preponderates. Water excess alone does not cause oedema (*see* pp. 8, 9). If a hyponatraemic patient appears clinically to be suffering from neither saline deficiency nor excess he is likely to have pure water excess and the most likely reason is 'inappropriate' secretion of ADH (*see* p. 29).

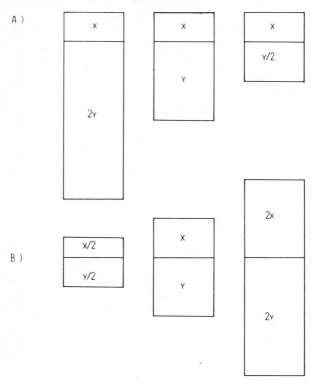

Fig 1.5 Variable interpretations of the plasma sodium concentration; X = the total amount of sodium in plasma; Y = the plasma water. A. Constant amount of sodium (X) but concentration changing because of varying water. B. Constant concentration of sodium but amount of both sodium and water changing.

WATER AND ELECTROLYTE BALANCE

In considering the likely extent of disturbance of body fluids it is useful to remember:

1. the range of usual intakes of water and electrolytes
2. the normal limits of excretion
3. the likely quantity and quality of abnormal losses through usual or unusual channels.

Range of Normal Intakes

'Normal' intake varies widely. The kidney, however, shows a remarkable degree of tolerance. Output normally adjusts rapidly to intake.

The customary ranges of intake of electrolytes and of protein are given in Table 1.6. National habit and individual appetite largely determine the salt intake; dietary protein is the major source of potassium.

Table 1.6
THE RANGE OF CUSTOMARY WATER, ELECTROLYTE AND
PROTEIN INTAKE IN W. EUROPE AND N. AMERICA

Sodium	90–180 mmol/24 h
Potassium	50–100
Calcium	5– 25
Magnesium	1– 4
Chloride	80–160
Phosphate	5– 25
Protein	60–180* g/24 h
Water	1– 4 l/24 h

* On the basis that 6 g of mixed protein contains about 1 g of nitrogen; the nitrogen intake range is therefore of the order of 10–30 g.

So effective is the kidney in excreting and conserving both water and electrolytes that only the most extreme variations are harmful.

Limits of Sodium, Potassium, and Water Conservation and Excretion

Urine, faeces and sweat are the only major normal routes of water and electrolyte excretion and expired air is the only source of pure water loss. The normal losses and the extent to which they can be reduced or increased by varying intake or external environment are outlined in Table 1.7. Intestinal excretion is largely independent of intake.

The kidney is the key to homeostasis in the face of constantly changing water and electrolyte intake.

Table 1.7
THE LIMITS OF SODIUM, POTASSIUM AND WATER
EXCRETION IN URINE, SWEAT AND FAECES
IN HEALTH

		Sodium *mmol/24 h*	*Potassium* *mmol/24 h*	*Water* *l/24 h*
Urine	min	1	10	0.25★
	usual	120	80	1.5
	max	>1500	>400	> 20§
Sweat	usual	25	5	0.5
	max	500†	100	10
				ml/24 h
Expired air	usual	—	—	0.1
	max	—	—	4‡
Faeces	min	1	10	50
	usual	5	20	120
	max	10	40	200

★ Depends upon the osmotic load to be excreted.
† The large sodium loss is a temporary phenomenon and is quickly reduced by acclimatisation. Potassium loss is not reduced.
‡ Highest losses in those with a tracheostomy.
§ If the increased fluid load is water without solute the limit is about 15 l/24 h (*see* p. 20).

Obligatory water loss has three components:

1. Respiratory and surface loss; at least 500 ml daily in a temperate climate
2. Faecal water – about 100 ml daily
3. Urine– sufficient water (1 l or more daily) to enable the daily electrolyte and urea load to be excreted in fluid of an osmolality within the maximum concentrating ability of the kidney.

Respiratory and surface loss increases several-fold with fever, in hot weather, as a consequence of heavy physical exertion and during hyperventilation. Respiratory water loss is substantially increased by tracheostomy. Severe diarrhoea increases faecal water loss to several litres daily.

An understanding of the relationship between protein intake and urea excretion is an important part of a working knowledge of body fluids because urea is the major source of urinary osmoles. In health, the urinary nitrogen output (less the 1 g or so of nitrogen lost in faeces) equals the dietary intake.

The following considerations and approximations provide necessary background information:

1. Urea ($CO(NH_2)_2$), which has a molecular weight of 60 and contains 2 atoms of nitrogen per molecule, is quantitatively the only important end product of protein catabolism; approximately one half ($\frac{28}{60}$) of urea molecule is nitrogen.
2. Since 6 g of protein contains approximately 1 g of nitrogen and 2 g of urea also contain approximately 1 g of nitrogen, 6 g of protein generate 2 g of urea, i.e. 1 g of urea is produced by 3 g of protein.

A diet containing 100 g of protein daily will therefore generate about 33.3 g of urea, an osmolar load of 555 mmol (mosmol) ($33.3 \times 1000/60$) on the kidney.

The maximum concentrating ability of the kidney determines the least amount of water required as solvent for the excretion of both the daily intake of electrolytes and the urea derived from protein metabolism. If water intake falls short of the minimum excretory requirement water is drawn from the total body water and water depletion ensues. The ability to concentrate the urine declines with increasing age; the maximal concentration is about 700 mmol (mosmol) in the elderly and 1200 mmol (mosmol) or higher in young adults.

The osmolar load provided by a diet containing 100 g of protein, 100 mmol of sodium and 70 mmol of potassium is as follows:

Sodium + anion (mainly chloride)	200 mmol (mosmol)
Potassium + anion (mainly chloride)	140 mmol
Urea	555 mmol
Total	895 mmol

The total load imposed by the diet is therefore within the osmolar content of 1 l of maximally concentrated urine. When insensible loss is about 500 ml a normal water intake of about 1.5 l is well judged.

A much larger water intake can be accommodated. The maximum diluting capacity of the kidney yields a urine with a concentration of about 70 mmol (mosmol). Thus even with a modest diet providing 700 mmol (mosmol), 10 l of maximally dilute urine could be excreted. A larger water intake would dilute body fluids.

Quantity and Quality of Abnormal Losses

Water and electrolyte therapy is best planned with knowledge of the order of abnormal losses. Whenever possible losses should be measured but fistulous discharge, in particular, may be difficult to collect. Daily weighing is a very useful guide to fluid balance, but is unfortunately difficult to achieve accurately in seriously ill patients, even with a weighing bed.

Fluid intake and output (including estimated losses when unmeasurable) must be charted as accurately as possible from day to day; each day's balance must be carefully noted and used to plan the next day's therapy. In any complex situation the cumulative fluid balance should be charted separately with an adjustment for estimated insensible loss.

The approximate composition of fluids lost in disease is given in Table 1.8.

The Value of Measurement of Urinary Electrolyte Excretion

Although water and electrolyte disturbances arise much more commonly from external imbalance than from internal redistribution, measurement of 24 h urinary excretion of electrolytes is generally of no value unless the intake is known and excretion by other normal and abnormal routes is measured.

Even when intake is defined and constant and there are no other losses than the small daily loss in faeces and sweat, the imbalance between intake and output may be so small as to be within the experimental errors of urinary collection and electrolyte measurement; the difference may, however, be sufficient as a cumulative imbalance to cause disease.

Only in a few extreme circumstances is measurement of urinary electrolyte concentration or 24 h excretion immediately

Table 1.8
THE COMPOSITION OF BODY FLUIDS LOST IN DISEASE

Ref‡		Na^+ mmol/l	K^+ mmol/l	Cl^- mmol/l	HCO_3^- mmol/l	H^+ mmol/l	Order of water loss ml/h
	Gastrointestinal						
1	Gastric juice pH 3	55	14	107	—	38	80–120
2	pH 6★	80	17	92	8	—	50
	Small intestine						
3	ileostomy (recent)	120	5–10	45			up to 120
4	ileostomy (adapted)	120	10–20	45			20
	Colon						
5	diarrhoea (severe)	100–130	10–20	80–100	30–50	—	up to 500
6	diarrhoea (mild)	100	10	90	20	—	up to 80
	villous adenoma	130	20	130	20	—	up to 80
7	congenital chloride losing diarrhoea	70	50	130	2	—	4–50
	Renal†						
	Diabetes insipidus	Concentration of electrolytes depends on urinary flow rate: no electrolyte losses attributable to diabetes insipidus *per se*					up to 600

★ Values depend on dilution of gastric juice by saliva. Pure specimens: Na^+ 137, K^+ 6, Cl^- 117, HCO_3^- 25 mmol/l.

† The electrolyte composition of urine in different forms of renal disease is too variable to be tabulated usefully here; the order of mismatch between intake and output of sodium and of potassium is considered in chapters 3 and 4.

‡ *See* numbers in Further Reading, p. 22.

informative. For example, a urinary concentration of potassium greater than 10 mmol in a hypokalaemic patient indicates failure of renal conservation (whether as a result of renal or adrenal disease); a urinary sodium concentration in an ECF-depleted patient greater than 20 mmol/l indicates impaired renal conservation of sodium.

Further Reading

Andersson B. (1977). Regulation of body fluids. *Ann. Rev. Physiol*; **39**:185–200.

Anonymous (1978). Hyponatraemia. *Lancet*; **i**:642–4.

De Wardener H.E. (1978). The control of sodium excretion. *Amer. J. Physiol*; **253**:F163–73.

[1] Documenta Geigy (1977). Scientific Tables, 8th edn. Basel.

Edelman I.S., Leibman J. (1959). Anatomy of body water and electrolytes. *Amer. J. Med*; **27**:256–77.

Feig P.U., McCurdy D.K. (1977). The hypertonic state. *N. Engl. J. Med*; **297**:1444–54.

[6] Fordtran I.S. (1967). Speculations on the pathogenesis of diarrhea. *Fed. Proc.*; **26**:1405–14.

[2] Gardham J.R.C., Hobsley M. (1970). The electrolytes of alkaline human gastric juice. *Clin. Sci.*; **39**:77–87.

[3] Goligher J.C. (1980). *Surgery of the Anus, Rectum and Colon*, 4th ed. London: Baillière Tindall.

Guyton A.C. (1978). Essential cardiovascular regulation – the control linkages between bodily needs and circulatory function. In *Developments in Cardiovascular Medicine* (Dickinson C.J., Marks J. eds.) pp. 265–302 Lancaster: MTP Press.

Harrington J.T., Cohen J.J. (1975). Measurement of urinary electrolytes – indications and limitations. *N. Engl. J. Med*; **293**:1241–3.

[7] Holmberg C., Perheentypa J., Launiala K., Hallman N. (1977). Congenital chloride diarrhoea. *Arch. Dis. Childh.*; **52**:255–67.

Leaf A. (1962). The clinical and physiologic significance of the serum sodium concentration. *N. Engl. J. Med*; **267**:24–30, 77–83.

Leaf A. (1970). Regulation of intracellular fluid volume and disease. *Amer. J. Med*; **49**:291–5.

Maxwell M.H., Kleeman C.H.R., eds (1972). *Clinical Disorders of Fluid and Electrolyte Metabolism*, 2nd edn. New York: McGraw-Hill.

[4] Nuguid T.P., Bacon H.E., Boutwell J. (1963). The ileostomy. *Dis. Colon. Rect.*; **6**:293–6.

Owen J.A., Edwards R.G., Coller B.A.W. (1970). *The Mole in Medicine and Biology*. Edinburgh: Livingstone.

5 Pierce N.F., Sack R.B., Mitra R.C., Banwell J.G., Brigham K.L., Fedson D.S., Mondal A. (1969). Replacement of water and electrolyte losses in cholera by an oral glucose-electrolyte solution. *Ann. Intern. Med.*; **70:**1173–81.

Pitts R.F. (1963). *Physiology of the Kidney and Body Fluids.* Chicago: Year Book Publishers.

Strickler E. M. (1966). Extracellular fluid volume and thirst. *Amer. J. Physiol*; **211:**232–8.

2.

Water

Thirst and antidiuretic hormone (ADH) are the keys to water balance. Thirst is normally controlled by plasma osmolality but thirst may also be stimulated by non-osmotic factors such as a fall in plasma volume (probably mediated by angiotensin) and be either stimulated or suppressed by hypothalamic disease.

Plasma osmolality also normally determines the release of ADH, although ADH is released in response to other stimuli such as pain, nicotine or a fall in plasma volume. The osmolality of plasma is monitored in the supraoptic nuclei of the hypothalamus (the 'osmostat') from which neurosecretory pathways pass to the posterior pituitary. The interrelationship between plasma osmolality and ADH-release are commonly disrupted in illness resulting in hyponatraemia, hypo-osmolality and plasma volume expansion (as in various situations of 'paradoxical' ADH-release, *see* p. 29).

Rarely, in the presence of hypothalamic disease, hypernatraemia and hyperosmolality occur without disturbance of plasma volume ('resetting the osmostat').

ADH controls the degree of waterproofing in the distal renal tubule, facilitating reabsorption of distal tubular fluid until the osmolality of the tubular fluid approaches that of the medulla. In the absence of ADH, distal tubular epithelium is almost impermeable to water and urine is very dilute. Water regulation may fail for a variety of reasons outlined in Table 2.1.

Total body water amounts to 50–70% of body weight in adults, varying inversely with the proportion of adipose tissue. For that reason the total body water is proportionately less in females than males. Water comprises 75–80% of body weight of infants who are especially vulnerable to disorders of water intake or loss for several reasons. The normal daily water intake of an infant is a much larger proportion of this total body water than in an adult; the ill-effects of both excess or deficient intake are magnified

Table 2.1
DISTURBANCES OF WATER REGULATION

DEFICIENCY
Deficient intake
{ 1. Inadequate water supply available
2. Failure of thirst to stimulate intake,
    e.g. coma
        hypothalamic lesions

Excessive output
{ 1. <u>Surface:</u> Increased evaporation
2. <u>Kidney:</u> Failure to concentrate urine,
    e.g. diabetes insipidus
    Osmotic diuresis without full water replacement, e.g. hyperosmolar diabetic coma, repeated mannitol or urea administration
    Other renal losses without full water replacement, e.g. polyuria after urinary tract obstruction or acute tubular necrosis.
3. <u>Intestine:</u> e.g. severe diarrhoea

EXCESS
Excessive intake
{ 1. <u>Therapeutic error</u>
2. Excessive drinking
3. Repeated hypotonic enemas
4. Water absorption during transurethral resection of the prostate

Reduced output
{ 1. Paradoxically concentrated urine
    ADH release in defence of plasma volume★
    Inappropriate ADH release in cerebral tumour, haemorrhage, infection, polyneuropathy, lung infections
    Ectopic ADH secretion by tumours
    Drugs with ADH-like activity or stimulating ADH release
    Other conditions: adrenal glucocorticoid deficiency, hypothyroidism
2. Renal failure

★ Water excess in this condition is more often relative than absolute

accordingly. The surface area of infants is much larger in proportion to body weight than in adults with a correspondingly increased susceptibility to skin water losses. Finally, the kidney does not achieve the ability of an adult to dilute the urine until about 2 weeks after birth and to concentrate until about 3 months; the relative inability to concentrate urine results from the small renal tubular urea load of a rapidly growing infant.

WATER DEFICIENCY

Hypernatraemia is the cardinal biochemical sign of selective water depletion, together with a raised plasma urea (partly as a result of increased haemoconcentration and partly as a result of a fall in urine flow).

Deficient Water Intake

Inadequate water supply

Shortage of water normally results from accident. But in hospital patients may become water depleted because they are unable to communicate their need.

Patients recovering from cerebrovascular accidents or from neurosurgery form the largest group at risk from an insufficient water intake especially if their tube feed provides a large osmolar load (*see* pp. 19, 153).

Failure of thirst

Thirst rarely fails in a conscious individual although it may be blunted by age. Unconscious patients can, of course, neither experience thirst nor control their intake and are entirely at the mercy of their medical attendants. Rarely, hypothalamic disease (usually a tumour) destroys the thirst-producing mechanism; such patients drink too little and become chronically dehydrated. Other patients with hypothalamic disturbance become hypernatremic without any evidence of water depletion, apparently as a result of a resetting of the hypothalamic 'osmostat'.

Excessive Water Output

Surface

Febrile patients, hyperventilating patients, patients with extensive burns and any individual in hot weather substantially increase their 'insensible' loss from skin and lungs from 600 ml to several litres per 24 h. It is easy to underestimate these losses. Unconscious patients and patients with burns or impending heat stroke are most at risk.

Kidney

The obligatory production of large volumes of very dilute urine (diabetes insipidus) is caused by a lack of ADH (for example after head injury) or by insensitivity of the kidney to ADH (renal diabetes insipidus). Both these circumstances are rare.

Urine more concentrated than plasma can, however, be formed without ADH if there is salt and water depletion. In these circumstances an increased proximal tubular reabsorption of sodium and a reduced GFR limit the volume of urine. In this way the induction of moderate ECF deficiency by administration of a thiazide diuretic paradoxically diminishes the urine volume of patients with diabetes insipidus.

In osmotic diuresis a pharmacologically inert plasma solute (glucose, mannitol etc.) is freely filtered at the glomerulus and undergoes limited tubular reabsorption. With high molar intratubular concentrations of the solute several factors contribute to the increased urine flow: dilution of sodium in proximal tubular fluid reduces sodium (and chloride) reabsorption and the isosmotic transfer of water which accompanies it; increased flow through the loop of Henle disturbs the countercurrent multiplier system; and increased delivery of water to the collecting duct reduces the maximum concentrating ability because more water is transferred from the collecting duct into interstitial fluid which is correspondingly diluted. The increased tubular flow rate also results in a clinically significant increase in urinary output of sodium and a smaller increase in potassium. Glucose causes an osmotic diuresis in uncontrolled diabetes mellitus, resulting in a depletion of water and, to a lesser extent, of sodium and potassium. The high plasma osmolality attracts intracellular water into plasma and accentuates the ICF deficit. Dehydration of the brain causes confusion, then coma – 'hyperosmolar' coma in contrast to the more usual acidotic diabetic coma due to keto-acids or lactic acid.

Intestine

Gastrointestinal fluids normally have a sodium concentration lower than plasma. Consequently patients become hypernatremic when there are extensive gastrointestinal losses unless the extra water loss is replaced.

WATER EXCESS

Water Excess due to Increased Intake

Therapeutic error

Excessive infusion of 5% dextrose or hypotonic saline is the commonest cause of selective water excess.

Excessive drinking

Rapid drinking of large volumes of hypotonic fluid is dangerous. Rapid dilution of plasma causes an osmotic shift of water into cells and acute overhydration of the brain, resulting in confusion, ataxia, convulsions and coma. Cold fluids may cause cardiac arrest through vagal stimulation. Which of these two hazards was the undoing of Grenadier Thomas Thatcher who died drinking cold beer on a hot day is anyone's guess. His tombstone by the West door of Winchester Cathedral offers both a warning –

> *'Soldiers be wise from his untimely fall,*
> *And when ye're hot, drink strong or none at all'*

and consolation –

> *'An honest soldier never is forgot,*
> *Whether he die by musket or by pot.'*

The plasma of heavy beer-drinkers may become persistently diluted to an extent sufficient to cause confusion, especially if they are malnourished. Plasma sodium concentrations as low as 98–107 mmol/l have been recorded in individuals habitually drinking 4–15 l of beer daily.

It is possible to drink water faster than it can be excreted. Water in gross excess can be as intoxicating as alcohol and is sometimes consumed for that reason:

Two psychopaths are on record who, after reading a newspaper article on the intoxicating effects of water addiction, embarked on a free binge. One gave up on account of severe headache while the other continued resolutely and developed convulsion and coma before he reached his target of 17 l.

These two patients recovered but it is a dangerous game with deaths on record from acute cerebral overhydration.

Reasons for excessive, persistent ('compulsive') water drinking include a fetish for inner cleansing and the elimination of imaginary parasites. The differential diagnosis of diabetes insipidus from compulsive water drinking is considered in Appendix B (p. 143).

Repeated hypotonic enemas

It is worth remembering that water intoxication can arise from rectal administration:

A 63-year-old man became constipated when recovering from a trans-urethral resection of his prostate. Two large soap-and-water enemas were given. Shortly after the second enema he became confused. His plasma sodium concentration was 107 mmol/l. Normally he would rapidly have excreted the water load, but in his postoperative condition he was unable to. He made a rapid recovery in response to water restriction. His name, Thursting, described the one thing which he was not! (It is possible that water absorbed during irrigation of his bladder after prostatectomy also contributed to his overhydration.)

Water Excess due to Reduced Output

Paradoxical concentration of urine

This group includes the syndrome of 'inappropriate' secretion of ADH associated with acute illness (especially intracerebral and pulmonary), ectopic ADH secretion, drugs exerting an ADH-like action and conditions such as adrenal glucocorticoid and thyroid deficiency. 'Inappropriate' implies that if the plasma osmolality is low, urine should be maximally dilute, or at least more dilute than plasma. Thus any situation in which plasma osmolality is low and urine osmolality exceeds plasma has for some time been considered to be an example of the syndrome of inappropriate ADH release. Urine can, however, become more concentrated than plasma without ADH (*see* p. 27) and it cannot be assumed that ADH is always responsible for a paradoxically concentrated urine.

The term 'inappropriate' also overlooks the fact that pain and trauma cause ADH release (postoperative pain is a major cause of reduced water excretion, body water expansion and hyponatraemia in surgical practice) and that the two major controllers of ADH-release may conflict, namely, a change in plasma osmolality and in effective plasma volume. The latter appears to be the stronger stimulus with the result that many seriously ill, ECF-depleted patients become hyponatremic, especially if they have been taking diuretics.

Patients with an expanded plasma volume as a result of excessive ADH secretion develop a sodium diuresis. The mechanism of this diuresis is uncertain: aldosterone secretion is not suppressed; altered intrarenal dynamics or a natriuretic hormone may prove to be responsible.

More readily available measurement of plasma ADH concentration may clarify the extent to which ADH is or is not responsible for the hyponatraemia of acute illness, although there will still be arguments as to the 'appropriateness' of any particular concentration in any particular situation. The important thing to remember is that symptoms are usually those of the associated illness and not attributable to hyponatraemia (at least above 120 mmol/l). Treatment of the underlying illness and water restriction usually corrects the hyponatreamia.

Most patients with initially unexplained hyponatraemia prove to have a carcinoma (usually an oat-cell carcinoma of the bronchus) which is secreting ADH-like peptides. The ectopic ADH syndrome was one of the most exciting medical discoveries of of the 1950s and has been the forerunner of a succession of ectopic hormone syndromes associated with malignant disease.

Diagnosis of this syndrome can be difficult, not least because of the intermittency and variety of cerebral symptoms.

A 53-year-old man suffering from headaches for several weeks decided one summer that he had been working too hard and needed a day at the seaside with his family. The train had not travelled far when he suddenly lost consciousness and had a convulsion. Two army medical orderlies incorrectly diagnosed cardiac arrest and began cardiac massage and mouth-to-mouth resuscitation.

When the train stopped at the next station an ambulance took him to the nearest hospital. By this time the patient was bruised but awake and unable to understand why he should not continue his journey.

Routine tests were sent and received routine inattention. After an overnight stay he was discharged and decided to make a second foray to the seaside. On this occasion he did not get quite so far down the line before he again had a convulsion and was taken to a different hospital.

Here he was deeply unconscious on arrival with a bizarre mixture of neurological signs. His plasma sodium was 102 mmol/l. Chest x-ray showed a bronchial carcinoma.

Several commonly used medicines such as chlorpropamide and carbamazepine have an ADH-like action, either by combining with ADH-receptors, or by stimulating ADH release or by lowering the level of plasma osmolality at which ADH is released (resetting the 'osmostat'). Although these drugs are commonly used, hyponatraemia is uncommon and is rarely sufficiently severe to cause symptoms.

Hyponatraemia is a common finding in patients with adrenal cortical deficiency because, without glucocorticoids, urinary dilution is imparied and without mineralocorticoids ECF volume is reduced and ADH is released. It is uncertain whether the occasional finding of hyponatraemia in hypothyroidism reflects a need for thyroid hormone to permit urinary dilution or whether ADH-release is abnormal.

Renal failure

Body fluids are diluted in acute renal failure if water intake and endogenous production exceeds the volume of urinary output and insensible water loss. The ability to excrete a water load is usually preserved in chronic renal failure until the preterminal stage of kidney disease.

Table 2.2 summarises the major causes of absolute or relative water excess with urine either more concentrated than plasma or less than maximally dilute. The Table includes sodium shifts, discussion of which has been postponed because of the uncertainties surrounding them.

Table 2.2

MAJOR CAUSES OF ABSOLUTE OR RELATIVE WATER EX-
CESS WITH URINE LESS THAN MAXIMALLY DILUTE IN
PRESENCE OF HYPONATRAEMIA

Absolute water excess
1. Intake excessive in relation to impaired renal function
2. Severe, chronic heart failure
3. ADH-release in response to acute illness or operation, especially
   intracranial and pulmonary disease
4. Ectopic ADH
5. Drugs promoting ADH action

Relative water excess
1. ADH-release to preserve ECF volume in combined salt and water
   deficiency (ADH release inappropriate in relation to plasma osmolality but appropriate in response to low plasma volume)
2. Sodium shift into cells

Relative Water Excess due to Sodium Shift into Cells

Hyponatraemia normally indicates a reduced plasma osmolality
due to dilution and not an exchange of sodium for other cations.
But as extrusion of sodium from cells depends upon an energy
dependent active transport system, it is reasonable to consider
whether in acute illness complicated by anoxia, hypothermia or
metabolic poisons, the sodium pump activity would be impaired
so that sodium accumulated in cells. For this reason, hyponatraemia in serious illness has sometimes been interpreted as the
result of a 'sick-cell syndrome'.

The reason for doubt concerns the osmotic consequences of a
shift of sodium into cells. If cell sodium increases, water should
move with it to preserve isotonicity of body fluids; alternatively
another cation must move in the opposite direction, or sodium
must become osmotically inactivated within the cells. But even if
sodium lost its osmotic activity by combining with polyvalent
anions, why should ECF remain hypotonic or, if it is hyponatremic but not hypotonic, what is the source and nature of the
additional osmoles? Even if some water has moved into cells
because of the fall in ECF osmolality, why is the relative excess of
plasma water not excreted by the kidney? Either ADH activity is
present in excess (in which case a sodium shift is no longer a

necessary part of the explanation) or, possibly, the 'osmostat' has been reset at a lower level as a consequence of altered intracellular composition. More information is needed before the truth is known.

Further Reading

Alford F.P., Scoggins B.A., Wharton C. (1973). Sympathetic normovolemic essential hypernatremia. *Amer. J. Med*; **54**:359–70.

Arieff A.I., Guisado R. (1976). Effects on the central nervous system of hypernatremic and hyponatremic states. *Kidney Int*; **10**:104–16.

Bartter F.C., Schwartz W.B. (1967). The syndrome of inappropriate secretion of antidiuretic hormone. *Amer. J. Med*; **42**:790–806.

Berl T., Anderson R.J., McDonald K.M., Schrier R.W. (1976). Clinical disorders of water metabolism. *Kidney Int*: **10**:117–32.

Fitzsimmons J.T. (1976). The physiological basis of thirst. *Kidney Int*; **10**:3–11.

Harrington J.T., Cohen J.J. (1973). Clinical disorders of urine concentration and dilution. *Arch. Int. Med*; **131**:810–32.

McDonald K.M., Miller P.D., Anderson R.J., Berl T., Schrier R.W. (1976). Hormonal control of renal water excretion. *Kidney Int*; **10**:38–45.

Morgan D.B., Thomas T.H. (1979). Water balance and hyponatraemia. *Clin. Sci*; **56**:523–32.

Robertson G.L., Shelton R.L., Athar S. (1976). The osmoregulation of vasopressin. *Kidney Int*; **10**:25–37.

3.

Sodium

Sodium intake is determined more by custom than by need. A usual British diet provides about 120 mmol of sodium daily. Blood pressure tends to be higher in people who take a large amount of sodium than in those who take little. This relationship is seen most clearly in some patients with chronic renal disease whose blood pressure can be controlled simply by restricting dietary sodium. A large salt intake predisposes to hypertension in genetically susceptible individuals but the extent to which the overall incidence of hypertension would fall if salt-intake were generally reduced is speculative.

Urinary excretion of sodium is tailored to the dietary intake; only about 100 mmol of the 25 000 mmol of sodium filtered daily in the glomeruli are excreted. The sites at which sodium is reabsorbed in the normal tubules are shown in Fig 3.1 together with the sites of action of common diuretics. Notes on the mechanisms involved are provided in Tables 3.1 and 3.2.

Total body sodium averages 60 mmol/kg of body weight but of this only 60% is readily exchangeable. The remainder is in bone, cartilage and dense connective tissue. The normal range of plasma sodium concentration is 135–145 mmol/l.

The major ways in which sodium regulation may break down in disease are summarised in Table 3.3.

SODIUM DEFICIENCY

Deficient Intake of Sodium

Renal conservation of sodium is normally so effective that it is difficult to induce symptomatic sodium deficiency by reducing intake. The kidney adjusts well to gradual reduction of sodium intake; abrupt and substantial reduction results in negative

34

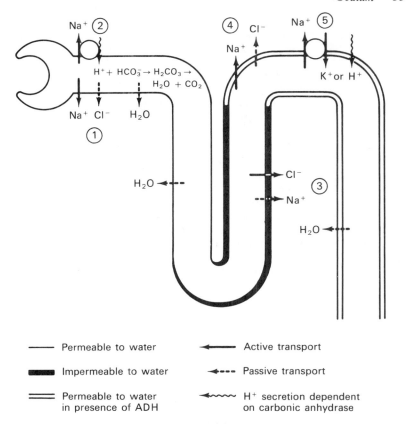

Fig 3.1 Sites of reabsorption of sodium in the kidney.

balance for two or three days before sodium excretion falls to
equal intake or to less than 5 mmol/day in total deprivation.
Vomiting not only prevents intake but is also a source of sodium
and water loss.

Excessive Output of Sodium

Kidney

Acute illness which does not involve the kidney may reduce the
renal excretory capacity for sodium but conditions in which the

Table 3.1

NOTES ON THE MAJOR SITES OF SODIUM REABSORPTION

Site (see Fig 3.1)	Mechanism	Proportion of total Na reabsorption
(1)	Active Na^+ reabsorption, Cl^- and H_2O follow: result, isosmotic reabsorption of NaCl.	70%
(2)	Active Na^+ reabsorption in exchange for H^+ which reacts with filtered HCO_3^- to form CO_2 and H_2O which are reabsorbed: regulation depends on generation of H^+ by tubular cells, dependent on carbonic anhydrase activity; result, reabsorption of $NaHCO_3$.	
(3)	Active Cl^- reabsorption, Na^+ follows: tubular fluid becomes hypotonic to plasma and interstitial fluid hypertonic; result, reabsorption of NaCl without H_2O – ability to concentrate urine (by countercurrent mechanism) depends on this function.	25%
(4)	Active Na^+ reabsorption, Cl^- follows: result, reabsorption of NaCl and water, tubular fluid becoming iso-osmotic with plasma if ADH active; in absence of ADH tubular fluid remains hypotonic – ability to dilute urine depends on this function.	
(5)	Active reabsorption of Na^+ in exchange for K^+ and H^+ dependent on aldosterone: balance between K^+ and H^+ as counter-ion depends partly on generation of H^+ in tubular cells, which is itself dependent on carbonic anhydrase.	5%

Table 3.2
SITES OF ACTION OF COMMON DIURETICS ON SODIUM
REABSORPTION

Type of diuretic	*Site of action* (Numbers refer to Fig 3.1)	*Examples*
Thiazide	Mainly site (4) but also site (1) (also weak carbonic anhydrase inhibitor so H^+ excretion at site (5) reduced and K^+ secretion increased; more Na^+ reaches this site and also favours K^+ loss).	Bendrofluazide Chlorothiazide Metolazone
Loop	Mainly site (3) but also site (4) (more Na^+ reaches site (5) increasing both K^+ and H^+ loss: hypo-kalaemia and alkalosis; inhibition of loop transport reduces corticomedullary osmotic gradient and therefore reduces ability to concentrate urine.)	Frusemide Bumetanide Ethacrynic acid
Possium-sparing	Site (5) Spironolactone by acting as competitive inhibitor of aldosterone	Spironolactone
	Other drugs by different mechanisms	Amiloride Triamterene
Carbonic anhydrase inhibitor	Sites (2) and (5) by diminishing availability of H^+ for exchange (weak action; used in treating glaucoma by reducing carbonic anhydrase-dependent secretion of aqueous humour).	Acetazolamide
Osmotic	Sites (1) – (5) non-specifically by maintaining large tubular volume by means of poorly reabsorbed small molecules (electrolyte reabsorption only slightly decreased per litre but volume of urine may be very large).	Mannitol Urea

Table 3.3
DISORDERS OF SODIUM METABOLISM IN DISEASE

DEFICIENCY	
Deficient intake	Inadequate supply <u>vomiting</u> starvation

Excessive output	1. Kidney
	   failure of sodium conservation in acute illness
	   chronic sodium-losing renal disease
	   adrenal cortical insufficiency
	   diuretics
	2. Intestine
	   <u>vomiting</u>
	   small intestinal fistula or recent ileostomy
	   chronic diarrhoea
	3. Surface (increased sweating)
	   heavy physical exertion
	   exposure to hot climate
	   <u>high fever in acute illness</u>

EXCESS	
Excessive intake	1. Therapeutic excess, usually i.v. 2. Unrecognised dietary sources in patients with impaired excretion.

Deficient output	1. Reduced renal perfusion,
	   e.g. <u>heart failure, hypoalbuminaemia</u>
	2. Renal failure: acute/chronic
	3. Acute glomerulonephritis
	4. Sodium-retaining hormones
	   hyperaldosteronism
	   cortisol excess
	   oestrogens and progesterone
	5. Sodium retaining drugs or food (*see* Table 3.5)
	6. Overcompensation to diuretic therapy

kidney is damaged by ischaemia or toxicity from either bacterial toxins or from drugs are more likely to impair conservation of sodium.

Patients with chronic renal disease neither conserve nor eliminate sodium normally. A very few patients with chronic renal tubular disease lose more sodium than any normal intake provides; the term 'sodium-losing renal disease' is sometimes applied only to this extreme end of the spectrum, but we use it more widely to focus attention on the inability of most patients with chronic renal disease to reduce their urinary sodium excretion rapidly in response to a lowered intake. The sodium intake of patients with chronic renal failure needs to be tailored to the often narrow band between their obligatory output and their upper limit of sodium excretion.

The serious consequences of a fall in sodium intake for a person who relies upon a large intake is illustrated by the following case, which also illustrates the ease with which the situation may be remedied:

> A 60-year-old man with large renal calculi gradually became unwell before starting to vomit several times each day. Figure 3.2 shows his rapid response to rehydration predominantly with isotonic saline. His blood urea fell promptly and a rise in weight of 5 kg indicated the extent of his initial fluid depletion.
>
> Subsequent measurement of his urine sodium loss on a defined intake showed that he needed a sodium intake of more than 120 mmol daily to avoid a deficit; when his intake was reduced to only 20 mmol daily his weight fell and renal function deteriorated judged from a rising blood urea (Fig 3.3). He was accordingly given a daily supplement of sodium chloride to ensure an intake of at least 120 mmol daily.

The approach to the use of a salt supplement in chronic renal failure is discussed further in Appendix B (*see* p. 133).

Urinary sodium and water losses are occasionally so large for several days after the relief of urinary tract obstruction that i.v. replacement is necessary.

Cortisol (hydrocortisone) regulates both carbohydrate and protein metabolism (glucocorticoid actions) and electrolyte excretion (mineralocorticoid actions); aldosterone has only mineralocorticoid effects. Both hormones are reduced in chronic adrenal cortical insufficiency (Addison's disease) and ECF is accordingly reduced. Selective aldosterone deficiency has been described in the elderly. Both the sodium and potassium effects of cortisol deficiency are discussed below (*see* p. 62) and the treatment of acute adrenal insufficiency (Addisonian crisis) can be found in Appendix B (p. 142).

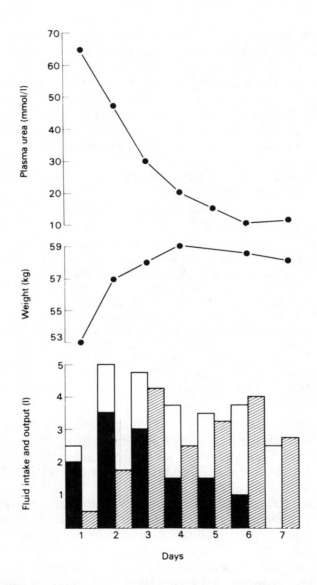

Fig 3.2 Fall of plasma urea, increase in urine output (▨) and increase in body weight of a 60-year-old man with acute-on-chronic renal failure caused by sodium losing renal disease who was rehydrated with isotonic saline (■) and other fluids (□). From Richards (1979) with permission of Blackwell Scientific Publications.

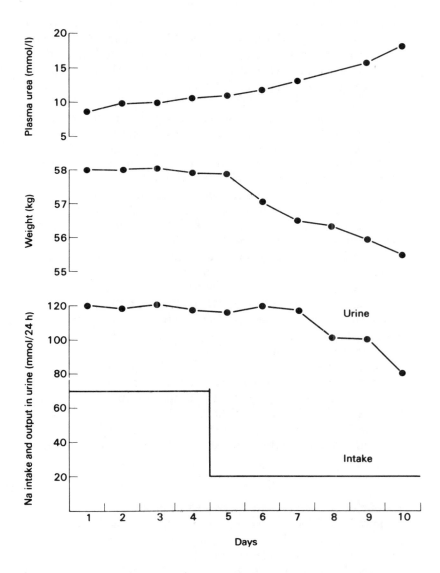

Fig 3.3 Obligatory urinary sodium loss substantially in excess of a low intake. *Note*: the failure to reduce urinary sodium loss in response to a 20 mmol intake until the cumulative salt and water deficit (reflected in loss of weight) was sufficient to decrease GFR (indicated by a rising plasma urea). From Richards (1979) with permission of Blackwell Scientific Publications.

Diuretics are a common cause of excessive renal excretion of sodium. The sites of action of diuretics are shown in Fig 3.1 and Table 3.1. Care must be taken to avoid excessive salt and water loss during diuretic therapy especially in the elderly. This is particularly difficult in severe chronic congestive heart failure where there is a narrow borderline between the beneficial and the harmful effects of plasma volume reduction. Excessive reduction of plasma volume may impair cardiac output and reduce GFR.

Concealed taking of diuretics is often both difficult to diagnose and difficult to treat. The patients are usually women who work in a paramedical profession or have medical relatives; hypokalaemia is usual and the plasma urate is usually raised (because most diuretics both reduce the renal tubular secretion and increase reabsorption of urate). The ill-effects of hypokalaemia usually predominate (*see* p. 52).

Elderly patients readily become confused and unwell when their plasma volume falls. Severe saline deficiency often induces vomiting which starts a vicious circle of increasing ECF depletion. So easy is it to over-treat with diuretics that it is a wise working rule that the elderly should not, except in acute left ventricular failure, be given a loop-diuretic in the first instance; a thiazide or a distal tubular diuretic (provided renal function is good) or a combination of the two should be used first.

Chronic diuretic treatment predisposes to hyponatraemia for several reasons. The degree of ECF reduction may be sufficient to activate ADH release. If plasma volume is severely reduced thirst is stimulated and saline losses are replaced by water. Also, diuretics themselves reduce the ability to form a dilute urine.

Intestine

ECF deficiency may be caused by loss of gastric, small intestinal or colonic fluid. The concentration of sodium is highest in small intestinal fluid (*see* Table 1.8) and losses from small bowel fistulae or an ileostomy are potentially the most serious. Vomiting wastes fluid with a lower sodium concentration but also prevents intake so that the negative balance rapidly increases. Although colonic fluid normally has a low sodium concentration, the more copious the diarrhoea the closer its composition approaches to small intestinal fluid.

Surface

Heavy physical work, prolonged exercise or exposure to hot climatic conditions all may cause sufficient salt and water loss through sweating to cause symptomatic saline depletion. Sweat may amount to several litres daily. Unaccustomed exposure to these conditions is dangerous; acclimatisation gradually and substantially reduces the losses of salt and to a lesser extent of water. Persons at risk need to take salt tablets and a liberal fluid intake. It is important to realise that salt loss from sweating in an acute febrile illness may be considerable. Sweat is always hypotonic to plasma with the result that excessive losses of sweat deplete both ECF and ICF but ECF is reduced to a relatively greater extent than if the losses had been of water only.

SODIUM EXCESS

Oedema is the cardinal sign of sodium excess (*see* p. 11). Plasma sodium concentration remains normal if plasma osmotic control operates normally. Table 3.4 outlines the major conditions associated with oedema.

Excessive Intake of Sodium

Therapeutic excess

Over-infusion with saline is the commonest cause of salt and water overload. The excess which can be tolerated without serious consequences depends partly on cardiac function and partly on the rate at which the saline is infused. Even when heart function is normal, rapid, massive saline infusion may cause heart failure; given slowly, much of the excess escapes into the interstitial space and causes oedema.

Appropriate fluid replacement may be particularly difficult to judge after major surgery with uncertain perioperative losses and a slow return of renal function.

Correct diagnosis and appropriate treatment can be difficult when a patient starts to pass apparently inexplicable large volumes of urine after operation but the most likely cause is a large input.

Table 3.4
PRINCIPAL CONDITIONS ASSOCIATED WITH
GENERALISED OEDEMA FORMATION

1. Increased central venous pressure:
    excessive sodium intake
    heart failure
    renal failure
    acute glomerulonephritis
    sodium-retaining drugs or foods
2. Reduced plasma albumin:
    increased loss: nephrotic syndrome
                         protein-losing gastroenteropathy
    reduced synthesis: chronic liver disease
3. Increased capillary permeability:
    vascular damage due to drugs, physical factors, or to local infection
    immunological capillary damage, e.g. serum-sickness
    'idiopathic' oedema
4. Mechanism uncertain:
    chronic respiratory disease without heart failure
    postimmobilisation

The following patient illustrates both a diagnostic pitfall and
the remarkable ability of the kidney to excrete an excessive load
of salt and water:

A 72-year-old man was recovering from an aorto-femoral bypass
graft. On the third postoperative day his urinary output marginally
exceeded his intake and his CVP measured between +1 and −2 cm;
his blood pressure was normal and he appeared to be well perfused.
In fact, had his cumulative fluid balance (excluding insensible loss)
been calculated he was 4.5 l in excess, so there was no cause for
concern.

The next day's output substantially exceeded intake in spite of an
increase of intake from 3 to 12 l but the difference was appropriate to
correction of the overall cumulative excess. Missing this important
point and considering instead the possibility of either pituitary or
renal diabetes insipidus associated with postoperative polyuric acute
tubular necrosis (both rather rare conditions) the house surgeon
increased the 24 h fluid intake to the remarkable figure of 26 l daily.
In that period the patient received 2354 mmol of sodium, 2244 mmol
of chloride, 135 mmol of bicarbonate, 225 mmol of lactate and

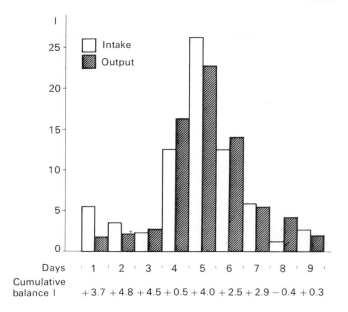

Fig 3.4 Fluid intake, urinary output and cumulative fluid balance (excluding insensible loss) in a 72-year-old man given excessively large postoperative fluid replacement.

250 mmol of potassium. A new complication, glycosuria due to the 570 g of glucose he received in the 26 l infusion, contributed to a fortuitous osmotic diuresis.

His intake was then reduced: Fig 3.4 shows that as his intake was reduced he corrected his overall cumulative balance. There was no evidence of an obligatory polyuria. Intake had been driving his output. It was unfortunately not feasible to weigh him during his illness.

Unrecognised oral intake

Oral intake is rarely a cause of sodium excess in individuals with normal renal function except in infants, whose ability to excrete sodium is very limited, but an occasional disturbed patient deliberately contrives to take sufficient salt to produce oedema. Unrecognised sources of sodium and sodium retaining medicines are easily overlooked; some are listed in Table 3.5.

Table 3.5
THE APPROXIMATE AMOUNT OF SODIUM PROVIDED BY
MEDICINES

Preparation	Sodium content	Sodium absorbed from likely max daily dose
*Antacids**	mmol/10 ml	mmol
Mag. carbonate BPC	10	60
Mag. trisilicate BPC	6	36
Aluminium hydroxide gel BPC	1	6
Mag. hydroxide BPC	< 0.1	< 1
Ion exchange resins	mmol/15 g	
Sodium polystyrene sulphonate ('Resonium A')	45	30–180†
Calcium polystyrene sulphonate ('Calcium Resonium')	< 0.1	< 1
Antibiotics	mmol/megaunit	
Benzyl penicillin-Na	2	20–40
	mmol/g	
Other penicillins	2–5	30–55
Carbenicillin		50–100

* Based on Barry R.E., Ford J. (1978). Sodium content and neutralising capacity of some commonly used antacids. *Brit. Med. J.*; **1**:413.
† The actual sodium load depends upon the amount of sodium exchanged for potassium, the remainder of the sodium being excreted in faeces bound to the resin.

Sodium-cycle ion exchange resins, which are used to reduce plasma potassium concentrations, are substantial sources of sodium. A normal daily dose of 45 g of sodium-cycle resin binds about 135 mmol of potassium and releases an equal amount of sodium, most of which is absorbed from the gut. An equivalent amount of calcium is released from a calcium-cycle resin but most of the calcium released is precipitated as calcium phosphate and is not absorbed. Calcium-cycle resins are therefore more suitable for use in renal failure.

Deficient Output of Sodium

Reduced renal perfusion

Reduced renal perfusion is a major factor in the pathogenesis of sodium (and water) retention associated with heart failure, nephrotic syndrome and chronic liver disease. Retained saline is lost into the interstitial space: in heart failure because of a raised venular capillary pressure and in nephrotic syndrome and chronic liver disease because of a low plasma oncotic pressure (*see* p. 13).

Acute or advanced chronic renal failure

Salt is always retained in acute renal failure but a normal dietary intake of sodium can be excreted by many patients with chronic renal failure until their disease is far advanced.

Sodium-retaining hormones

Aldosterone and cortisol cause salt and water retention; aldosterone has a far greater effect weight for weight. In primary mineralocorticoid excess, the kidney escapes from the sodium-retaining action of these hormones after the retention of 3–4 l of saline before oedema develops. Hypertension is usual. The plasma sodium concentration is normal or slightly raised; plasma renin activity and angiotensin concentration are low and suppressed. When, however, excessive secretion of aldosterone is secondary, i.e. part of a continuing compensatory mechanism as in heart failure, hypoalbuminaemia or repeated vomiting, sodium and water retention continues, the blood pressure is normal or low and the plasma sodium concentration is usually low-normal or low, plasma renin activity and angiotensin concentration are raised.

Oestrogens and to a lesser extent progesterone are sodium-retaining, their effects being seen most commonly in premenstrual oedema. Sodium retention associated with their therapeutic use is discussed below.

Sodium-retaining drugs or foods

Drugs promote sodium retention either indirectly by lowering blood pressure or by a direct renal tubular action (Table 3.6). All

Table 3.6
SODIUM-RETAINING PREPARATIONS

1. Mediated by fall in blood pressure:
     all hypotensive drugs
2. Direct renal action even without fall in blood pressure:
     diazoxide
3. Mediated by mineralocorticoid action:
     licorice
     carbenoxolone
     cortisone and related steroids
4. Probably mediated by reduction in renal prostaglandin synthesis:
     phenylbutazone, indomethacin, and other
     non-steroidal anti-inflammatory drugs
5. Mediation uncertain:
     monoamine oxidase inhibitors
     oestrogens and progesterone

drugs which effectively lower blood pressure induce sodium retention as a homeostatic response to reduced perfusion pressure in the kidney. Vasodilators such as diazoxide are the most potent sodium-retainers regardless of whether or not systemic blood pressure is reduced. Diuretics are given simultaneously with hypotensive drugs partly to avoid saline retention, partly because they have a mild vasodilator action of their own and also because they lower blood pressure by reducing plasma volume.

Licorice and carbenoxolone have a structure and action on the distal renal tubule similar to aldosterone and may cause severe oedema and hypokalaemia.

Many non-steroidal anti-inflammatory and analgesic drugs cause salt and water retention, as may monoamine oxidase inhibitors. Both groups of drugs should not be given to patients particularly at risk from ECF expansion.

A small proportion of women taking oestrogen/progesterone mixtures for contraception, especially tablets in which oestrogens predominate, develop oedema. Oestrogens remain standard treatment for carcinoma of the prostate; large doses have not proved superior to small and the larger the dose the greater the risk of heart failure from plasma volume increase.

A temporary rebound of salt and water retention is usual and may be alarming when prolonged diuretic treatment is stopped. Nevertheless, it is generally in the patient's best interest to ride out the storm even when, as in the following case, the rebound is disturbing:

> A 31-year-old female patient was inappropriately treated with frusemide for six months. Within two days of stopping she noticed ankle oedema and within 10 days she had gained 7 kg and was passing little urine. Her JVP was raised and she had moderate oedema. Without treatment she lost the excess fluid over the next 10 days.

Further Reading

Anderson R.J., Linas S.L. (1978). Sodium depletion states. Sodium and water homeostasis. In *Contemporary Issues in Nephrology*, vol. 1. (Brenner B.M., Stein J.H. eds.). New York: Churchill-Livingstone.

Anonymous (1969). Vomiting. *Lancet*; i:142–3.

Levy M. (1978). The pathophysiology of sodium balance. *Hospital Practice*; **13**:95–106 (11).

Richards P. (1979). Conservative management of chronic renal failure. In *Clinical Medicine and Therapeutics* (Richards P., Mahler H., eds), pp. 127–37. Oxford: Blackwell Scientific.

Swales J.D. (1975). *Sodium Metabolism in Disease*. London: Lloyd-Luke.

4.

Potassium

Potassium, the major intracellular cation, is both essential to the action of many intracellular enzymes and contributes to the electrical potential difference across cell membranes by the ratio of its concentrations in ECF (3.5–5.0 mmol) and ICF (160 mmol). The resting potential determines the ease with which muscular contraction is initiated and a normal plasma potassium concentration is necessary for normal cardiac contraction and re-polarisation. Total body potassium, which is closely related to muscle mass, averages 42 mmol/kg of body weight in adults. Although total plasma potassium normally accounts for only 0.4% of total body potassium, changes in plasma potassium concentrations generally reliably reflect changes in body potassium.

About 100 mmol of potassium are normally taken daily, mainly in protein. Potassium intake cannot easily be reduced below 40 mmol daily. Obligatory losses amount to about 20 mmol daily of which about half is lost in faeces and half in urine. Potassium filtered in the glomerulus is reabsorbed in the proximal tubule; some is secreted in the distal tubule in the exchange of postassium and hydrogen ion for sodium which is controlled by adrenal mineralocorticoids (*see* p. 36).

As much potassium can be excreted in health as is ingested in all but the most unusual circumstances. A raised plasma potassium concentration stimulates the secretion of aldosterone and therefore increases excretion of potassium and hydrogen ion in exchange for sodium in the distal renal tubule; aldosterone also increases the colonic secretion of potassium.

Intravenous administration opens the door to excess undreamt by nature and care must be taken neither to give too much nor to infuse too rapidly, especially to those with poor renal function. Potassium should not be infused at a rate exceeding 40 mmol/h or in a concentration greater than 40 mmol/l; bolus injections should *never* be given of potassium from stock ampoules (containing for example 26 mmol in 20 ml). The dosage of potassium must take account of muscle mass and plasma potassium concentration must be determined frequently in patients receiving i.v. supplements. A daily potassium maintenance dose of 78 mmol (6 g of potassium chloride) is both sufficient and safe for patients receiving only i.v. fluids provided there are no unusual losses and renal function is normal.

The concentration of potassium in plasma has to be interpreted with knowledge of several possible reasons for a spuriously high concentration *in vitro*. For example, the plasma potassium concentration rises because of a potassium leak from muscle if blood is taken after prolonged venous compression and especially if the arm is exercised in order to increase venous return. The net effect is insufficient to cause hyperkalaemia but it may conceal hypokalaemia. The concentration of potassium in serum is 5–10% higher than in plasma due to platelet consumption during coagulation.

Traumatisation of red cells in the course of a difficult venepuncture causes haemolysis with release of red cell potassium into plasma, especially if the plasma is not separated from the cells quickly. It should, however, never be assumed that hyperkalaemia reported on a haemolysed specimen is due to haemolysis. The patient may be hyperkalaemic as a result of acute intravascular haemolysis or a cause unrelated to the haemolysis. A fresh specimen should be taken carefully and analysed at once.

A rare inherited erythrocyte potassium leak is of occasional diagnostic importance. Such patients appear to have alarmingly high plasma potassium concentrations unless blood samples are centrifuged and separated immediately after venepuncture; their erythrocytes do not leak potassium *in vivo*.

A very high platelet count causes spurious hyperkalaemia in serum because platelets leak potassium in the process of coagulation. Abnormal leukocytes in leukaemia may also leak potassium *in vitro* during coagulation.

Plasma potassium concentration is not always an adequate guide to overall potassium balance because shifts of potassium may develop between ECF and ICF (*see* p. 63).

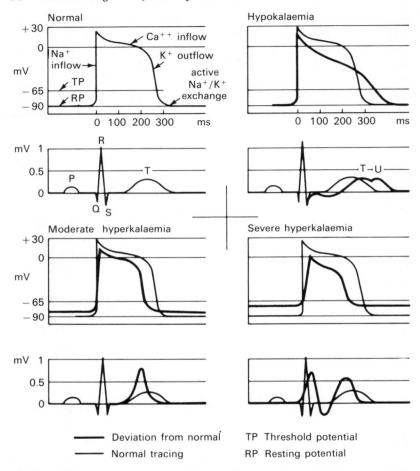

Fig 4.1 The electrocardiogram in hypo- and hyperkalaemia. (From Welt L.G. (1975). Regulation of the intracellular environment. In *The Sea Within Us* (Bricker N.S., ed.) p. 29. San Juan: Searle & Co.)

SYMPTOMS AND SIGNS OF POTASSIUM DEFICIENCY AND EXCESS

Hypokalaemia causes muscle weakness, sometimes sufficiently profound to cause paralysis. Severely hypokalaemic patients also have nocturia partly because the kidneys fail to concentrate the urine maximally and partly because the normal diurnal rhythm of sodium and water diuresis during the day is reversed. Reversal of this diurnal rhythm is a non-specific feature of many illnesses but is often pronounced in hypokalaemia. The disorder of repolarisation of muscle characteristic of hypokalaemia is reflected in the presence of U waves on the electrocardiogram (ECG) (Fig. 4.1) and in progressive disturbances of heart function (Table 4.1).

Table 4.1
THE ECG ABNORMALITIES ASSOCIATED WITH HYPOKA-
LAEMIA IN USUAL ORDER OF PROGRESSION

1. U waves
2. Disappearance of T wave into U wave
3. Widening of QRS complex
4. Dysrhythmias
    ventricular extrasystoles
    supraventricular tachycardia
    nodal tachycardia
    ventricular tachycardia
    ventricular fibrillation

Hyperkalaemia is symptomless until extreme (over 8 mmol/l), when it causes weakness and extreme mental agitation. Disorders of heart rate and rhythm develop before symptoms (Fig 4.1 and Table 4.2); ventricular fibrillation or standstill is the final and fatal cardiac manifestation of hyperkalaemia.

Table 4.2
THE ECG ABNORMALITIES ASSOCIATED WITH HYPERKA-
LAEMIA IN USUAL ORDER OF PROGRESSION

1. T wave peaking
2. ST-segment increasingly acute
3. Atrio-ventricular block
4. P wave diminution then disappearance (atrial standstill)
5. Widening of QRS complex (interventricular block)
6. QT prolongation
7. Dysrhythmias
    ventricular tachycardia
    ventricular fibrillation
    ventricular standstill

The more rapid a disturbance of potassium the more likely it is to be symptomatic. Extreme hypokalaemia (under 2 mmol/l) may be asymptomatic if it develops slowly. Patients may survive plasma potassium concentrations as low as 1.2 mmol/l and as high as 9 mmol/l, but such deviations are dangerous.

POTASSIUM DEFICIENCY

Table 4.3 summarises the major conditions in which potassium regulation is disturbed.

Table 4.3
DISORDERS OF POTASSIUM METABOLISM IN DISEASE

DEFICIENCY

Deficient intake
1. Starvation
2. Repeated vomiting

Excessive output

(a) *Renal*
1. Diuretics (osmotic, thiazide, loop or acetazolamide)
2. Osmotic diuresis
   heavy glycosuria
   mannitol
3. Tubular disease
   renal tubular acidosis
   other tubular syndromes
   chronic pyelonephritis

(b) *Intestinal*
1. Diarrhoea
   acute gastroenteritis; cholera
   inflammatory bowel disease
   purgative addiction
   osmotic diarrhoea
   villous adenoma of colon
2. Malabsorption
3. Urinary diversion

cont'd opposite

Table 4.3 *cont'd*

Excessive
output
(cont'd)
	(c) *Renal and intestinal associated with*
	    mineralocorticoid excess
	1. Aldosterone
	    primary (Conn's syndrome)
	    secondary
	2. Carbenoxolone or licorice
	3. Cortisol (Cushing's syndrome)

EXCESS

Excessive *intake*	1. Oral 2. Parenteral
Reduced *output*	1. Inappropriate use of potassium-sparing diuretics 2. Acute or terminal chronic renal failure 3. Adrenal mineralocorticoid deficiency

SHIFTS

(a) ECF→ICF	1. Alkalosis 2. Insulin-induced 3. Carbohydrate-induced 4. Periodic hypokalaemic paralysis
(b) ICF→ECF	1. Acidosis 2. Acute intravascular haemolysis 3. Crush injuries 4. Depolarisation-blocking agents 5. Digitalis intoxication 6. Periodic hyperkalaemic paralysis

Deficient Intake

Starvation or repeated vomiting

Potassium is conserved less effectively than sodium. Consequently, starvation more readily results in potassium than sodium depletion. Repeated vomiting may result in potassium deficiency by preventing intake and, indirectly, by increasing loss. The potassium loss in vomit is small but the chloride loss in gastric juice is large. Chloride deficiency prevents renal conservation of potassium because proximal tubular reabsorption of sodium becomes limited by relative unavailability of chloride in the proximal tubule and more sodium reaches the distal tubule where it is reabsorbed in exchange for potassium and hydrogen ion. Distal tubular exchange is also stimulated by aldosterone secreted in this situation in response to sodium deficiency. Increased distal tubular exchange of sodium for potassium and continuing loss of hydrogen ion in gastric juice perpetuate both alkalosis and hypokalaemia. Only when the sodium deficiency is corrected and sufficient chloride is given to restore proximal tubular sodium reabsorption to normal can the potassium deficiency and alkalosis finally be corrected.

Correct interpretation of hypokalaemia may be long delayed when vomiting is concealed; misdiagnosis may even result in unnecessary surgery as the following case shows:

> A 15-year-old boy disliked both his work as a bricklayer's apprentice and his workmates who teased him for being fat. He became depressed and resentful, his appetite declined and he started to vomit. A correct diagnosis of psychogenic vomiting was made but he did not cooperate with psychiatric treatment.
>
> A few months later he visited another hospital with painful cramp in his hands and feet ('tetany') on account of extreme alkalosis (plasma bicarbonate 52 mmol/l). His blood urea was raised (10.6 mmol/l, 64 mg/dl) because he was dehydrated. He was hyponatraemic (122 mmol/l) and hypokalaemic (2.1 mmol/l); his plasma calcium was normal. All these abnormalities were corrected by i.v. saline and potassium chloride but soon returned when he was ambulant. It was noted that he ate little but he was not seen to vomit.
>
> When investigations revealed no abnormality of stomach or kidneys an incorrect diagnosis of primary hyperaldosteronism was made and an operation arranged to search for an adrenal tumour. This diagnosis failed to account for the fact that his blood pressure was low, his plasma renin high and that he had lost weight – the opposite of the findings in primary hyperaldosteronism.
>
> No tumour was found at operation. Subsequent investigation confirmed that he was vomiting surreptitiously.

Excessive Renal Output

Diuretics

Any diuretic with its major site of action proximal to the distal tubule increases potassium loss by inducing a mild salt deficiency (which stimulates secondary hyperaldosteronism) and also by flooding the distal tubule with sodium not absorbed proximally. The need to give potassium supplements to patients taking a diuretic is discussed in Appendix A (p. 120).

A very modest dose of diuretic even when given with a potassium supplement may cause profound illness, especially in the elderly as the following case illustrates:

> An 88-year-old man with heart failure had for several years taken a small dose of a thiazide diuretic and potassium in a combined tablet. His doctor sent him to hospital because he had become too weak to look after himself at home. The plasma potassium concentration was only 1.2 mmol/l. Dietary assessment showed that his habitual dietary potassium intake was only about 45 mmol daily.

It is clear that a routine small potassium supplement is no insurance against severe hypokalaemia.

The diagnosis of diuretic-induced hypokalaemia is difficult only in patients who deliberately conceal their diuretic-taking. Often they take diuretics in an attempt to slim, usually without being stout at the start. Sometimes concealed medication is a deliberate attempt (usually by a doctor's relative, a nurse or a pharmacist) to attract attention. Detection of a diuretic in the urine is the most convincing evidence but a raised plasma urate is also a useful pointer.

Osmotic diuresis

Potassium and sodium losses may be substantial in the osmotic diuresis generated by, for example, glycosuria in diabetes or following repeated doses of mannitol.

Tubular disease

Chronic metabolic acidosis caused by a discrete renal tubular inability to maintain the usually high hydrogen ion gradient across distal tubular epithelium (distal renal tubular acidosis) is associated with potassium deficiency, indeed the condition sometimes presents as hypokalaemic paralysis. There are several reasons for the potassium deficiency. Some patients have impaired sodium reabsorption and develop secondary hyperaldosteronism. Potassium metabolism is restored to normal in others when their acidosis is corrected. A few patients are not improved by either of these manoeuvres and it seems that their potassium deficiency results from a limitation in hydrogen ion availability in the distal tubular exchange of sodium for potassium and hydrogen ions.

Excessive urinary potassium loss is an occasional feature of a wide variety of chronic renal diseases, usually those with an obstructive or interstitial pathology.

Excessive Intestinal Output

Diarrhoea

Diarrhoea causes potassium depletion. Diarrhoeal stool is usually intermediate in composition between small intestine fluid (which has a high sodium and low potassium concentration) and normal stool (which has a low sodium and high potassium concentration) and a combined deficiency of both potassium and sodium is therefore common.

Purgative abuse is often difficult to diagnose. These patients are obsessed with the desirability of at least one daily bowel motion for inner cleansing. They often present with weakness resulting from potassium depletion. Sometimes they deliberately conceal their purgative-taking.

The urge to purge is old and has even become a political pawn. Rhubarb was one of the medicines denied to France by Britain during the Napoleonic Wars, an unworthy act of war on which Sydney Smith seized in his inimical way:

> 'What a sublime thought that no purge can now be taken between the Weser and the Garonne; that the busting pestle is still, the canonous mortar mute, and the bowels of man locked up for fourteen degrees of latitude. When, I should be curious to know, were all the powers of crudity and flatulence fully explained to His Majesty's ministers? At what period was this great plan of conquest and constipation fully developed?'

Examination of the stool by the doctor is an essential part of diagnosis. The diarrhoeal stool of one such patient smelled strongly of hydrogen sulphide, leading to a search of her possessions and the discovery of crystals of magnesium sulphate in a bottle labelled 'Bath salts'. Phenolphthalein-containing purgatives can be detected by the red colour obtained when sodium hydroxide is added to the stool. Chronic purgative abuse is dangerous and sometimes lethal, especially in patients with anorexia who not only eat little but may take both diuretics and purgatives. This is the worst of all worlds.

Some purgatives, such as sodium sulphate, act by causing an osmotic diarrhoea, sulphate being poorly absorbed. Intestinal lactase deficiency and sucrose-isomaltase deficiency, may cause an osmotic diarrhoea, partly by unabsorbed disaccharides attracting water into the small intestine and partly by the increase in osmotically active small molecules resulting from bacterial fermentation of disaccharides in the colon.

Congenital chloride-losing diarrhoea, a rare cause of osmotic diarrhoea, results from a defect in chloride absorption and both increases intestinal potassium loss and impairs renal conservation of potassium by inducing chloride depletion. Increased renin release in response to salt and water loss causes secondary hyperaldosteronism which further increases both renal and intestinal potassium loss.

A villous adenoma of the rectum may secrete sufficiently large volumes of watery mucus rich in sodium, potassium and chloride to cause serious deficiency of all three ions, with development of metabolic alkalosis (*see* p. 106). The sodium concentration of the fluids is usually a little below plasma, the chloride slightly above plasma concentration. The potassium concentration is very variable, but sometimes as high as 120 mmol/l.

Malabsorption

Small intestine malabsorption (as a result of either intestinal disease or pancreatic deficiency) may both impair potassium absorption and increase intestinal loss because of a fatty-acid induced osmotic diarrhoea. It is important to realise that by no means all such patients have diarrhoea. Muscle weakness due to potassium deficiency may be the presenting symptom, as in the case of a 40-year-old shop assistant who became unable to lift boxes up on the shelves.

Urinary diversion

The practice of transplanting ureters into the sigmoid colon to bypass bladder or bilateral lower ureteric disease has largely been replaced by the fashioning of a separate ileal conduit opening in a small stoma. Both operations may cause hypokalaemia and acidosis. Hypokalaemia results from increased sodium-for-potassium exchange in the bowel (especially the colon) in response to the urine flooding into it; hyperchloraemic acidosis results from reabsorption of chloride in exchange for bicarbonate secreted by the intestinal mucosa.

Excessive Renal and Intestinal Output

Aldosterone-excess

Hypokalaemia is the hall-mark of aldosterone excess, either primary, caused by an adrenal cortical adenoma or by multi-nodular hyperplasia, or secondary in response to activation of the renin/angiotensin system. Aldosterone stimulates sodium-for-potassium exchange in both distal renal tubule and in the colon. Primary hyperaldosteronism causes hypertension. Cases of primary hyperaldosteronism are seldom as clear-cut as the following example. The syndrome is important if uncommon because it is one of the few curable causes of hypertension.

A 28-year-old nurse suffered episodes of profound muscular weakness lasting up to about one day. For a few months she had had to pass urine several times each night (*see* p. 52).

Her blood pressure was 230/130 but her urine did not contain protein; her plasma urea was normal. She was hypokalaemic (1.8 mmol/l), hypernatraemic (147 mmol/l) and alkalotic (plasma bicarbonate 34 mmol/l). She excreted 40 mmol of potassium in her urine daily in spite of profound hypokalaemia (*see* p. 22).

Her plasma renin concentration was very low and did not rise in response to sodium deprivation; plasma aldosterone was raised. She was cured by the excision of an adrenal cortical adenoma.

Carbenoxolone and licorice

Carbenoxolone and licorice stimulate reabsorption of sodium in the distal tubule in exchange for potassium and hydrogen ion with the result that they cause hypokalaemia and alkalosis. Treatment with carbenoxolone may have serious consequences, especially if potassium-losing diuretics are used to reduce the oedema produced:

> A 70-year-old man was readmitted to hospital with weakness, dyspnoea and oedema four weeks after beginning treatment with carbenoxolone for a gastric ulcer. Subsequently he had visited his doctor on account of increasing oedema and breathlessness. Digoxin and a loop-diuretic (frusemide) were prescribed. He became profoundly weak with a plasma potassium of 2.2 mmol/l and developed a digoxin-induced irregularity of heart rhythm, because hypokalaemia potentiates digoxin. The disturbance of his cardiac function and the profound sodium and water retention induced by carbenoxolone more than offset the benefit of the diuretic and when admitted to hospital he weighed 20 kg more than when he had left hospital.

Cortisol excess (Cushing's syndrome)

Cortisol (hydrocortisone) has relatively weak mineralocorticoid actions compared to aldosterone. It is unusual in Cushing's syndrome caused by adrenal hyperplasia or adenoma for the degree of mineralocorticoid excess to be sufficient to cause more than a marginal rise in plasma sodium and fall in potassium; moderate hypertension is usual but oedema is rare. Electrolyte upset is minimised in treatment with adrenal corticosteroids by the use of prednisolone.

When, however, Cushing's syndrome is caused by an adrenal carcinoma or by the ectopic production of ACTH-like peptides (commonly from an oat-cell bronchial carcinoma) the degree of cortisol excess is sufficiently great to cause hypokalaemia. So rapid is the development of the syndrome that Cushingoid changes in body appearance usually have not had time to develop by the time hypokalaemia becomes symptomatic.

POTASSIUM EXCESS

Excessive Intake

Hyperkalaemia rarely arises from excessive intake if renal function is normal, although it has happened in unusual circumstances such as when a chronic alcoholic drank large volumes of a potassium elixir containing 4% alcohol.

Reduced Output

Inappropriate use of distal tubular diuretics

The administration of potassium supplements, distal tubular diuretics or both to patients with impaired renal function is an avoidable cause of potassium excess. Mixtures of diuretics should not be given without a clear understanding of the site of action and dose of the component drugs. Potassium supplements and distal tubular diuretics should never normally be given together although the combination has a place for a limited period in certain circumstances of potassium depletion.

Renal function should be assessed before a diuretic is given and be reviewed from time to time in case it should deteriorate during treatment.

Renal failure

The restriction and reduction of potassium in patients with renal failure is discussed in Appendix B (pp. 131, 133).

Chronic adrenal insufficiency (Addison's disease)

Addison's disease is rare but important because it is eminently treatable yet easily missed (especially in individuals who do not develop increased pigmentation). The onset of vomiting is a serious threat to a patient who is already saline-depleted and hyperkalaemic:

> A 43-year-old Spanish hospital domestic was admitted to a surgical ward having lost 7 kg in 2 months during which time she had felt generally unwell; recently she had begun to vomit.
>
> Being naturally swarthy in complexion it was difficult to assess the significance of her pigmentation but she had patchy pigmentation in her mouth as well as having deeply pigmented skin creases. Her lying blood pressure was low (85/65) and fell lower still on standing. She looked ECF-depleted.
>
> She had a high plasma potassium (6.2 mmol/l), low sodium (121 mmol/l), low bicarbonate (16 mmol/l) and high urea (18 mmol/l).

Her plasma cortisol was very low both at 9 am and at midnight and hardly increased at all after an injection of a synthetic analogue of ACTH. Plasma ACTH measurement was not available at the time but would have shown a very high concentration. An x-ray of her abdomen showed fine calcification of both adrenal glands characteristic of tuberculosis.

Within 5 days of starting treatment with i.v. isotonic saline, cortisone and fludrocortisone her fluid and electrolyte balance had been corrected.

Suspicion of the correct diagnosis is often slowly aroused in the absence of pigmentation. The plasma electrolytes may be normal. Biochemical confirmation is not usually difficult once the diagnosis is suspected. Patients operated upon for the unexplained abdominal pain, which is a frequent symptom, or for an unconnected surgical illness are especially at risk because they cannot respond normally to stress; they may become gravely hypotensive and develop an 'Addisonian crisis' (Appendix B p. 142).

POTASSIUM SHIFTS

Intracellular potassium concentration is maintained at its high level by a combination of electric and osmotic forces. The sodium/potassium pump ensures the rapid removal of sodium from cells. The large amounts of organic anion in cells (mainly protein and phosphate) retain potassium in cells by electric forces against the concentration gradient.

Potassium concentration is about 30 times higher within cells than in plasma. A small percentage shift of intracellular potassium to ECF causes serious hyperkalaemia, while movement of a similar percentage of plasma potassium in the opposite direction makes little mark on the intracellular concentration.

ECF→ICF

Alkalosis

Potassium moves into cells in exchange for hydrogen ion whenever the plasma pH rises. One consequence is that hypokalaemia associated with persistent alkalosis is difficult to correct before the alkalosis itself is corrected.

Insulin and carbohydrate-induced

In both these situations glucose and potassium move into cells under the influence of insulin; the difference lies only in the inducing factor. Insulin, given with glucose to prevent hypoglycaemia, is used therapeutically to treat hyperkalaemia (*see* Appendix A p. 119). In the treatment of diabetes with insulin the intracellular movement of potassium is less welcome; indeed hypokalaemia is the most serious hazard of the treatment of uncontrolled diabetes. Similarly the provision of large amounts of carbohydrate orally or parenterally especially to patients previously deprived of carbohydrate, provokes a large insulin output and a shift of potassium into cells.

Familial periodic hypokalaemic paralysis

There are many uncertainties about this condition and its mirror-image, familial periodic hyperkalaemia, conditions in which episodic muscle weakness is associated with either hyper- or hypokalaemia which is not explained by changes in external balance. The evidence that potassium shifts are responsible for the electrophysiological changes in muscle is incomplete and the technical difficulties in obtaining such evidence are formidable.

ICF→ECF

Acidosis

Acidosis is buffered partly intracellularly by the replacement of potassium with hydrogen ion. If, as often happens in uncontrolled diabetes mellitus, external potassium losses are simultaneously increased, the paradoxical situation may develop in which plasma potassium is normal or even raised in spite of an overall total body deficiency. In this situation plasma potassium concentration may fall precipitously when insulin is given or the metabolic acidosis is rapidly corrected with bicarbonate.

Other causes

Several other causes of hyperkalaemia due to an acute shift of potassium into the ECF are listed in Table 4.3.

Conversely, hyponatraemia is sometimes interpreted as a sign of potassium deficiency, on the presumption that sodium replaced potassium within the cells. Whether this interpretation is ever true seems doubtful and, at least, awaits verification.

Further Reading

Brown J.J., Fraser R., Lever A.F., Robertson J.I.S. (1972). Aldosterone: physiological and pathophysiological variations in man. In *Clinics in Endocrinology and Metabolism* (Mason A.S., ed.) pp. 397–449. London: Saunders.

Cohen J.J. (1979). Disorders of potassium balance. *Hospital Practice*; **14**:119–28.

Cummings J.H., Sladen G.E., James O.F.W., Sarner M., Misiewicz J.J. (1974). Laxative-induced diarrhoea: a continuing clinical problem. *Brit. Med J*; **1**:537–41.

Giebisch G., Stanton B. (1979). Potassium transport in the nephron. *Ann. Rev. Physiol*; **41**:241–56.

Katz F.H., Eckert R.C., Gebott M.D. (1972). Hypokalaemia caused by surreptitious self-administration of diuretics. *Ann. Intern. Med*; **76**:85–90.

Schultze R.G. (1973). Recent advances in the physiology and pathophysiology of potassium excretion. *Arch. Int. Med*; **131**:885–97.

Schwartz W.B., van Ypersele de Strihou Ch., Kassirer J.P. (1968). Role of anions in metabolic alkalosis and potassium deficiency. *N. Engl. J. Med*; **279**:630–9.

Wallace M., Richards P., Chesser E., Wrong O. M. (1968). Persistent alkalosis and hypokalaemia caused by surreptitious vomiting. *Quart. J. Med*; **37**:577–88.

5.

Calcium

Calcium resembles potassium to the extent that its physiological effects depend primarily upon its concentration in ECF. The plasma concentration is, however, a poor guide to calcium balance because a normal ECF concentration may be maintained at the expense of bone. A high plasma calcium indicates either overall excess or excessive mobilisation.

Calcium helps to maintain the stability and excitability of cell membranes. Deviations in the calcium concentration of ECF alter the excitability of peripheral nerves, the central nervous system, skeletal, smooth and cardiac muscle: hypocalcaemia increases neuromuscular excitability and hypercalcaemia reduces it.

INTERPRETATION OF PLASMA CALCIUM CONCENTRATION

Protein-binding of Plasma Calcium

Only the ionised fraction of plasma calcium is physiologically important: normally 50–60% of the total plasma calcium is ionised (Table 5.1); a small proportion is complexed and the remainder is bound to plasma proteins, predominantly albumin. Ionisation of calcium is inversely proportional to the plasma pH. Consequently associated with hypocalcaemia chronic renal failure rarely causes symptoms because the patient is acidotic. Conversely, reduced ionisation of calcium in acute respiratory alkalosis (e.g. hyperventilation by an anxious patient) increases neuromuscular excitability, notwithstanding a normal total calcium.

Table 5.1
THE NORMAL COMPONENTS OF TOTAL PLASMA CALCIUM

		mmol/l
Ionised		1.35
Complexed		0.25
(with bicarbonate, citrate and phosphate)		
Protein-bound		0.90
to albumin 0.7		
to globulin 0.2		———
	Total	2.50

Note: to convert these values to mg/dl multiply by 4.

Correction of Total Plasma Calcium

Interpretation of total plasma calcium concentration requires correction for plasma protein. The protein-bound calcium depends on the plasma albumin. An albumin concentration of 40 g/l is taken as the appropriate reference point for many current, automated methods. For every 1 g/l by which the plasma albumin exceeds (or is less than) 40 g/l 0.02 is subtracted (or added) to the total plasma calcium expressed in mmol/l.

HYPERCALCAEMIA

Symptoms and Signs

Hypercalcaemia is commonly symptomless; routine screening has shown that symptomatic hypercalcaemia is only the tip of an iceberg. The major signs and symptoms are listed in Table 5.2; some of these, such as corneal calcification, radiologically apparent nephrocalcinosis, and renal calculi require months or years of hypercalcaemia; both nephrocalcinosis and renal calculi can also (and, in the case of renal calculi, more commonly do) result from hypercalciuria without hypercalcaemia. Symptoms of hypercalcaemia are proportional to its severity, the rapidity of onset and the duration.

Table 5.2
SYMPTOMS AND SIGNS OF HYPERCALCAEMIA

1. None or non-specific ill-health
2. Neurological and psychiatric
    Headache, lethargy, confusion
    Any psychiatric disturbance, including depression,
        hallucinations and paranoia
    Muscle weakness
3. Renal
    Nocturia, polyuria, increased thirst
    Nephrocalcinosis and/or renal calculi
    Renal failure
4. Gastrointestinal
    Dyspepsia with or without peptic ulceration
    Constipation
    Vomiting, difficulty in swallowing
    Acute pancreatitis
5. Dermatological
    Itching
    Skin ulceration
6. Ocular
    Corneal calcification
7. Cardiovascular
    ECG changes: short QT interval
    Hypertension
    Vascular calcification
8. Other tissues
    Calcium deposits

Causes of Hypercalcaemia
(Table 5.3)

Increased intestinal absorption of calcium

Excessive vitamin D intake
Hypercalcaemia is a substantial hazard of pharmacological doses
of calciferol (1.25 mg, 50 000 units or more daily) but may
develop on a near physiological dose; the normal daily requirement of an adult is 2.5 μg, 100 units, and the weakest BP
preparation of calcium and vitamin D contains 12.5 μg, 500 units
per tablet.

Table 5.3
MAJOR CAUSES OF HYPERCALCAEMIA

Increased intestinal absorption	1. Excessive vitamin D – treatment of rickets, osteomalacia, hypoparathyroidism and renal osteodystrophy 2. Increased sensitivity to vitamin D – sarcoidosis and infantile hypercalcaemia 3. Excessive calcium intake – milk-alkali syndrome 4. Hyperparathyroidism (minor component of its action)
Increased mobilisation	1. Hyperparathyroidism 2. Ectopic PTH secretion by carcinoma 3. Bone destruction by metastases or multiple myeloma 4. Prostaglandins and osteolysins from malignant tumour 5. Prolonged immobilisation 6. Recovery phase of acute renal failure 7. Thyrotoxicosis 8. Vitamin D excess (minor component of its action)
Decreased excretion	Thiazide diuretics
Mechanism uncertain	Adrenal cortical insufficiency

All patients treated with vitamin D must have their plasma calcium determined frequently. Prolonged hypercalcaemia may cause irreversible renal failure. A short acting analogue of vitamin D, such as 1α-hydroxycholecalciferol (alfacalcidol) has the advantage that overdosage is rapidly reversed on stopping treatment. On the other hand, the effects of vitamin D overdosage can rapidly be corrected with prednisolone, often by as little as 10 mg daily. Treatment may need to be continued for up to three months because calciferol and its metabolites are stored in liver and tissue lipids. Conversely, hypercalcaemia may take several months to develop on a fixed dosage of vitamin D.

Increased sensitivity to vitamin D

Patients with sarcoidosis and infants with idiopathic hypercalcaemia are excessively sensitive to vitamin D. Hypercalcaemia may only develop when another factor supervenes, such as increased synthesis of ergocalciferol in the skin in response to summer sunlight. Correction of a combination of relatively minor circumstances may enable treatment with adrenal corticosteroids to be avoided.

> An 84-year-old lady with dyspnoea due to pulmonary infiltration proved on liver biopsy to have sarcoidosis. Her plasma calcium initially was 2.80 mmol/l. She had for a few months been drinking 1 l of milk daily and taking a mutivitamin tablet, which contained a very small amount of calciferol (10 μg, 400 units). Stopping the vitamin tablet and the milk was sufficient intervention to allow her calcium to return to normal.

Although vitamin D excess causes hypercalcaemia predominantly by increasing intestinal absorption of calcium it also to a small extent mobilises calcium from bone.

Excessive calcium intake

A large calcium intake rarely by itself causes hypercalcaemia because the efficiency of absorption falls as the intake rises; at a normal intake of 800 mg (20 mmol) of calcium the efficiency of absorption is only 10–20%. Very large doses of absorbable calcium salts (usually calcium carbonate) and/or milk (which supplies 30 mmol of calcium per litre) cause hypercalcaemia in the 'milk-alkali'-syndrome. It is particularly disastrous when the thirst associated with hypercalcaemia is quenched with large volumes of milk as the following case shows:

> A 62-year-old man who had suffered from occasional renal colic for 24 years became increasingly thirsty and developed epigastric pain, occasional vomiting, flatulence and constipation. His doctor told him to stop drinking alcohol so he took to cold milk instead – up to 5 l daily.
> He was subsequently found to have a very high plasma calcium of 4.6 mmol/l (18.7 mg/dl), alkaline phosphatase four times the upper limit of normal and poor renal function. His plasma parathormone concentration was more than 10 times the upper limit of normal and X-rays of his bones showed characteristic subperiosteal bone resorption and lytic lesions of severe hyperparathyroid bone disease. He

was quickly admitted for the excision of a parathyroid tumour. On the first postoperative day he developed a severe acute pancreatitis (*see* p. 68) from which he died.

Prolonged use of a calcium-cycle ion exchange resin to control hyperkalaemia (*see* Appendix A (pp. 119, 133)) rarely causes hypercalcaemia, and probably only in those patients who have advanced secondary hyperparathyroidism.

Increased mobilisation of calcium

Hyperparathyroidism

Primary hyperparathyroidism as a result of a parathyroid adenoma or, rarely, a carcinoma is the commonest cause of hypercalcaemia in adults. Secondary hyperparathyrodism, parathyroid hyperplasia in response to prolonged hypocalcaemia or hyperphosphataemia, does no more than restore the plasma calcium to normal. Occasionally one or more of the hyperplastic parathyroids becomes autonomous and hypercalcaemia develops as a result of this 'tertiary' hyperparathyroidism. Hypercalcaemia is usually not severe in primary hyperparathyroidism (about 2.75–3.25 mmol/l, 11–13 mg/dl).

Renal failure is the most predictable complication of hypercalcaemia. GFR falls, proximal tubular reabsorption of sodium diminishes and the distal tubule becomes relatively unresponsive to ADH. Nocturia, polyuria and thirst are the initial symptoms as a recent case reminded us:

A 70-year-old woman was admitted with recent confusion and disorientation and a record of several months' ill health. She was drinking repeatedly from an imaginary cup as a token of her unslaked thirst. Her plasma calcium was 3.50 mmol/l. A large parathyroid adenoma was excised. After operation she developed acute pancreatitis from which she made a good recovery.

Ectopic parathormone secretion

Parathormone-like polypeptides may be secreted by a variety of malignant tumours of which the commonest is squamous carcinoma of the bronchus. Although parathormone and similar tumour polypeptides predominantly raise plasma calcium by mobilising calcium from bone, they also increase the intestinal absorption of calcium.

Bone destruction by metastases and multiple myeloma; prostaglandins and osteolysins from malignant tumours

Malignant tumours most commonly cause hypercalcaemia by bone destruction. Some, however, secrete prostaglandins which indirectly mobilise calcium either by stimulating osteoclasts directly or by inducing circulating monocytes to release an osteoclast-activating factor. Osteolysins may also be secreted by malignant tumours and act directly on bone producing a chemotactic substance which attracts tumour cells to areas of osteoclastic activity; the tumour cells either reabsorb bone directly or by stimulating osteoclastic activity.

Prolonged immobilisation

Prolonged immobilisation has fortunately become a rare facet of both medical and orthopaedic treatment. Patients particularly at risk during immobilisation are those with increased bone turnover as a result of Paget's disease or with an increased tendency to osteoporosis on account of treatment with adrenal corticosteroids. Previously the treatment of bone tuberculosis by bed rest and vitamin D was a frequent cause of hypercalcaemia, renal calculi and renal failure.

Recovery phase of acute renal failure

The plasma calcium usually falls precipitately in acute renal failure and may rebound to a hypercalcaemic level during recovery (*see* Appendix B, p. 132). It is important to wait a few days to allow time for a return to normal before concluding that hypercalcaemia preceded renal failure.

Thyrotoxicosis

Hypercalcaemia is an uncommon consequence of increased bone turnover in thyrotoxicosis. Very occasionally an associated parathyroid adenoma has been the cause of hypercalcaemia.

HYPOCALCAEMIA

Hypocalcaemia is frequently symptomless until an increased demand is made on calcium resources as in pregnancy.

Symptoms and Signs
(Table 5.4)

Table 5.4
SYMPTOMS AND SIGNS OF HYPOCALCAEMIA

1. None or non-specific ill-health
2. Neurological and psychiatric
   Tetany – overt or latent
   Convulsions
   Spinal cord disturbance
   Anxiety or depression
   Intracranial calcification in region of basal ganglia
3. Ocular
   Cataract
   Papilloedema
4. Gastrointestinal
   Abdominal pain
5. Dermatological
   Brittle, deformed nails
   Rashes: eczema; worsening of psoriasis
   Alopecia
6. Respiratory
   Recurrent laryngeal spasms
7. Cardiac
   ECG changes: prolonged QT interval

Diagnosis is simple if attacks of tetany (carpopedal spasms) occur. The feet are only occasionally involved. Sometimes less specific tightening or cramp is experienced in muscles after use (*see* p. 75). Ischaemia produced by inflating a sphygmomanometer cuff around the arm to a pressure just above the arterial pressure for not longer than 3–4 min may provoke tetany (Trousseau's sign). Firm percussion over the facial nerve anterior to the external auditory meatus may provoke twitching of the angle of the mouth (Chvostek's sign).

One of the rarest signs, papilloedema, is perhaps the most important because of the ease with which it can be misinterpreted in a patient with signs of cerebral disturbance. The pathogenesis of papilloedema in association with hypocalcaemia or of basal ganglia calcification (which is not necessarily associated with papilloedema) is obscure. Both signs are probably confined to those with chronic hypocalcaemia arising from idiopathic hypoparathyroidism.

Causes of Hypocalcaemia
(Table 5.5)

Table 5.5
MAJOR CAUSES OF HYPOCALCAEMIA

Deficient intake and/or absorption of calcium and vitamin D	1. <u>poor dietary intake</u> 2. <u>malabsorption</u> 3. postgastrectomy
Vitamin-D resistance	1. chronic metabolic acidosis: renal tubular acidosis 2. <u>chronic acidosis and uraemia</u>: <u>chronic renal failure</u>
Altered metabolism of vitamin D	liver-enzyme-inducing drugs e.g. phenytoin barbiturates
Deficient absorption and mobilisation of calcium	Hypoparathyroidism post-thyroidectomy idiopathic pseudohypoparathyroidism
Deficient absorption and mobilisation of calcium and increased deposition in bone	After excision of a parathyroid adenoma or total parathyroidectomy

Low intake of calcium, vitamin D or both

Poor dietary intake
Gone are the days of widespread vitamin D deficiency amongst children in the cities of Europe but dark-skinned immigrant children and their mothers (if they have repeated pregnancies) are very much at risk. Not only are they little exposed to sunlight (and therefore synthesise little ergosterol in their skin), but they are liable to have either a vegetarian diet, a generally poor diet or to eat chupati which bind calcium in the gut.

Malabsorption syndromes

Hypocalcaemia is one of a number of nutritional consequences of intestinal malabsorption. If, however, the degree of overall malabsorption is mild, hypocalcaemia may only develop if the vitamin D intake is marginal (remembering that vitamin D absorption is also diminished). In these circumstances diagnosis may be long delayed:

A 30-year-old Irishman, with the bearded appearance of James Galway and a liking for playing the recorder but not the flute, was seen recently complaining of feeling tired for seven or eight years; he was employed sweeping the streets by night. He did, however, mention that he had given up playing tennis because his legs and arms rapidly became very tired, that his tongue and lips were difficult to move after playing his recorder for long periods, and that his hands occasionally became stiff and uncomfortable. He denied any intestinal disturbance though he later recalled some diarrhoea in childhood. His diet was marginally deficient in vitamin D.

His plasma calcium was very low (1.24 mmol/l, 5.0 mg/dl) and the alkaline phosphatase was raised. His haemoglobin and plasma potassium were normal. Tests of intestinal absorption were abnormal. A bone biopsy showed osteomalacia and a jejunal biopsy showed the characteristic flat appearance of a gluten-sensitive enteropathy.

Partial gastrectomy

Malabsorption of calcium and vitamin D is common after partial gastrectomy but osteomalacia and hypocalcaemia do not normally develop until several years later, if at all.

Vitamin D resistance

Persistent metabolic acidosis either without general renal insufficiency, as in renal tubular acidosis, or as a feature of chronic renal failure, interferes with the action of vitamin D on both intestine and bone. Hypocalcaemia is more common than osteomalacia in chronic renal failure and the reverse is paradoxically true of renal tubular acidosis.

Resistance to the action of vitamin D is also found in patients with a renal tubular phosphate leak. Although they may develop osteomalacia, they do not normally become hypocalcaemic.

Altered metabolism of vitamin D

Drugs such as phenytoin and barbiturates accelerate the metabolism of vitamin D in the liver by enzyme-induction and reduce its effectiveness. In patients whose intake is marginal, especially growing children and elderly patients taking a poor diet, this alteration in the metabolism of vitamin D may tip a precarious balance in the direction of deficiency.

Deficient absorption and mobilisation of calcium

Hypoparathyroidism
Idiopathic hypoparathyroidism may present at any age but more commonly in childhood; the symptoms and signs are those of chronic hypocalcaemia (Table 5.4). A congenital insensitivity to parathormone (pseudohypoparathyroidism) may cause confusion.

Thyroidectomy is the commonest cause of hypoparathyroidism, but whether because of excision or ischaemic damage remains uncertain. Transient hypocalcaemia after thyroidectomy may sometimes be explained by deposition of calcium in bone when the rapid turnover characteristic of thyrotoxic bone disease is abruptly interrupted. Symptomatic hypocalcaemia may develop several years after thyroidectomy if vitamin D intake falls or new demands are made on body stores.

Deficient absorption and mobilisation of calcium with increased deposition in bone

After the excision of a parathyroid adenoma plasma calcium falls precipitously both because the other parathyroids have been temporarily suppressed by the autonomous hypersecretion of parathormone by the adenoma and partly because associated bone disease rapidly begins to heal. A similar but more severe situation is seen after total parathyroidectomy (*see* Appendix A (p. 123)).

Further Reading
Deftos L.J., Neer R. (1974). Medical management of the hypercalcaemia of malignancy. *Ann. Rev. Med*; **25**:323–31.

Epstein F.H. (1968). Calcium and the kidney. *Amer. J. Med*; **45**:700–14.

Habener J.F., Mahaffey J.A. (1978). Osteomalacia and disorders of vitamin D metabolism. *Ann. Rev. Med*; **29**:327–42.

Massry S.G., Friedler R.M., Coburn J.W. (1973). The physiology of the renal excretion of phosphate and calcium and its relation to clinical medicine. *Arch. Int. Med*; **131**: 828–59.

Schneider A.B., Sherwood L.M. (1975). Pathogenesis and management of hypoparathyroidism and other hypocalcemic disorders. *Metabolism*; **24**: 871–98.

6.

Magnesium

Magnesium is relatively unexplored in human disease. While it is an important activator of several cellular enzyme systems, it remains controversial whether deficiency of magnesium by itself causes symptoms. In general, a low plasma magnesium increases neuromuscular activity and a high concentration has the reverse effect, also depressing CNS function sufficiently to suppress convulsions and induce narcosis. The plasma concentration reflects excess more reliably than deficiency. Approximately 50% of plasma magnesium is protein bound.

MAGNESIUM DEFICIENCY

Hypomagnesaemia is so commonly associated with hypocalcaemia and hypokalaemia that it is difficult to discern its individual ill-effects. It has been both asserted and denied that hypomagnesaemia causes tetany indistinguishable from hypocalcaemic or alkalotic tetany; what does seem certain is that it may be impossible to control tetany adequately in a patient who is both hypocalcaemic and hypomagnesaemic until the plasma concentrations of both cations are restored to normal (*see* Appendix A (p. 123)).

The major causes of magnesium deficiency are listed in Table 6.1. A magnesium supplement is only required for postparathyroidectomy, severe malabsorption or malnutrition and prolonged i.v. feeding.

MAGNESIUM EXCESS

Magnesium is no longer used therapeutically to depress cerebral function. Retention of magnesium may contribute to nervous system depression in advanced renal failure.

Table 6.1
MAJOR CAUSES OF MAGNESIUM DEFICIENCY

1. Gastrointestinal	Malabsorption
	Malnutrition, especially alcoholics
2. Endocrine	Hyperparathyroidism, especially after excision of an adenoma
	Hypoparathyroidism
	Hyperaldosteronism
3. Prolonged diuretic therapy	
4. Prolonged i.v. feeding	

Further Reading

Anonymous (1976). Magnesium deficiency. *Lancet*; **i**:523–4.

Rude R.K., Singer F.R. (1981). Magnesium deficiency and excess. *Ann. Rev. Med*; **32**:245–9.

Wacker W.E.C., Parisi A.F. (1968). Magnesium metabolism. *N. Engl. J. Med*; **278**:712–7, 772–6.

7.

Phosphorus

The skeleton contains about 85% of total body phosphorus (amounting to 700–800 g); the remainder has an important structural and physiological role in cell membranes (phospholipids), nucleic acids, phosphoproteins, high-energy phosphates such as ATP and 2,3-diphosphoglyceric acid (2,3-DPG), and a variety of enzymes, co-factors and biochemical intermediates. Most diets contain sufficient phosphate to maintain adequate phosphorus stores and plasma phosphate concentration (0.71–1.36 mmol/l, 2.2–4.2 mg/dl); 85–90% of phosphate filtered at the glomerulus undergoes tubular reabsorption. On an intake of 1 g daily 700–800 mg of phosphate is excreted in urine and 200–300 mg in faeces.

Maintenance of phosphorus balance and a normal serum phosphate concentration depends on

1. adequate absorption of phosphate from the gastrointestinal tract,
2. well adjusted urinary phosphate excretion, and
3. a normal distribution of phosphate in the body.

HYPERPHOSPHATAEMIA

Table 7.1 lists the main causes of hyperphosphataemia. An acute decrease in renal phosphate excretion or an increase in absorptive capacity alone rarely increases plasma phosphate sufficiently to matter. Chronic renal failure is accompanied by hyperphosphataemia which, although not symptomatic itself, needs treatment to prevent secondary hyperparathyroidism (*see* Appendix B p. 134)). In contrast, exogenous phosphate loads, with or without pre-existing renal failure, may cause an abrupt and massive elevation of plasma phosphate concentration resulting in

80

Table 7.1
MAJOR CAUSES OF HYPERPHOSPHATAEMIA

Increased supply or absorption	Increased exogenous phosphorus load: oral orthophosphate medication phosphate infusions (treatment of hypercalcaemia) phosphorus burns (skin and gastrointestinal) Increased phosphorus absorption: vitamin D intoxication
Extracellular shift	Endogenous phosphate load: increased catabolism (e.g. in starvation) acute tissue breakdown (e.g. rapid response to therapy in malignant lymphoma and acute lymphoblastic leukaemia)
Decreased excretion	Decreased renal phosphate excretion: acute and chronic renal failure hypoparathyroidism and pseudohypoparathyroidism acromegaly, thyrotoxicosis, vitamin D intoxication

secondary hypocalcaemia due to calcium phosphate precipitation. Calcium phosphate is deposited in many tissues including the lungs, the myocardium and blood vessels; deposition in the kidney causes renal failure which worsens the patient's prognosis.

Treatment of massive, acute hyperphosphataemia includes the reduction of intake and endogenous load, reduction of absorption by means of oral phosphate binding antacids and even haemodialysis.

HYPOPHOSPHATAEMIA

Serious hypophosphataemia, a phosphorus concentration below 0.32 mmol/l (1 mg/dl) is either due to a decrease in intestinal phosphorus absorption, to an increased intestinal or renal phosphate loss, or to acute shifts of phosphate from the extracellular to the intracellular compartment (Table 7.2).

Severe phosphate depletion can cause signs and symptoms in

Table 7.2
MAJOR CAUSES OF HYPOPHOSPHATAEMIA

Reduced supply or absorption	alcoholism phosphate-binding antacids malabsorption/malnutrition prolonged vomiting/diarrhoea vitamin D deficiency/resistance
Increased renal loss	proximal tubular defects diuretics (prolonged large dosage) primary hyperparathyroidism
Intracellular shift	total parenteral nutrition treated ketoacidosis severe burns (recovery phase)

almost any organ system (Table 7.3). Most seem to result from a deficiency of ATP and/or 2,3-DPG, impairing either the cellular energy resources or the delivery of oxygen to the tissue.

Table 7.3
SYMPTOMS AND SIGNS OF PHOSPHATE DEPLETION

1. None or non-specific ill-health
2. Neurological and psychiatric:
     confusion
     convulsions
     coma
     intention tremor and/or ataxia
     cranial nerve palsies
     peripheral neuropathy
3. Skeletal muscle:
     weakness
     rhabdomyolysis
4. Bone:
     rickets/osteomalacia
5. Heart failure
6. Haemolysis
7. Renal:
     hypercalciuria
     glycosuria
     bicarbonate loss→metabolic acidosis

Further Reading

Fitzgerald F. (1978). Clinical hypophosphatemia. *Ann. Rev. Med*; **29**:177–89.

Knochel J.P. (1977). The pathophysiology and clinical characteristics of severe hypophosphatemia. *Arch. Int. Med*; **137**:203–20.

Lentz R.D., Brown B.M., Kjellstrand C.M. (1978). Treatment of severe hypophosphatemia. *Ann. Int. Med*; **89**:941–4.

Stoff J.S. (1982). Phosphate homeostasis and hypophosphataemia. *Amer. J. Med*; **72**:489–94.

8.

Urea and Creatinine

Neither urea nor creatinine are electrolytes but both are useful in the assessment of fluid balance. The plasma urea concentration is a convenient indicator of GFR; on an ordinary protein intake plasma urea is inversely proportional to urea clearance and urea clearance is directly proportional to GFR.

The clearance of urea $(\frac{UV}{P})$ at normal urine flow (>2 ml/min) is about half the GFR because of back-diffusion of urea from the renal collecting duct. At slower flow rates, as in dehydration or heart failure, backdiffusion increases and the plasma urea rises out of proportion to the fall in GFR. Conversely, at high urine flows urea is washed out from the renal medulla and the plasma urea falls without an increase in GFR.

The relationship between GFR and urea (and creatinine) is such that the plasma concentration rises little until the GFR falls to about 40% of normal (Fig 8.1). The plasma urea concentration

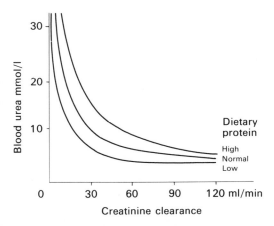

Fig 8.1 The relationship between blood urea concentration and creatinine clearance showing the effect of high, normal and low protein intakes.

84

also reflects protein intake. On a large protein intake the plasma urea is relatively high in relation to GFR (Fig 8.1) and the converse applies on a low protein intake. High protein intakes do not cause an appreciable increase in plasma urea if renal function is normal until the intake exceeds 2.5 g of protein/kg of body weight. A habitually much larger consumption of protein causes persistent azotaemia sufficient for the unwary observer to diagnose renal failure, as the following example illustrates:

> A thin 43-year-old woman was found at intervals over a period of 3 years to have a plasma urea persistently in the range of 22–30 mmol/l (132–180 mg/100 ml) although her plasma creatinine (and creatinine clearance) was normal. Her haemoglobin was also normal. She had no symptoms and was clearly azotaemic but not uraemic. At university 25 years previously she had developed anorexia nervosa; she learned to avoid criticism for not eating while yet remaining thin by eating large quantities of protein with practically no carbohydrate and little fat. Consequently, for 25 years she had eaten about 400 g of protein daily (9 g/kg body weight); at the time of investigation her diet comprised 'Casilan' (a low sodium protein powder derived from milk), cauliflower, cabbage and cod – except on Mondays when her fishmonger was closed and she ate meat.

The use of the plasma urea concentration as an index of GFR not only assumes a normal protein and fluid intake, but it also assumes nitrogen balance. Clearly, acute catabolic disease, for example after severe trauma or burns, may unload a sudden surge of urea into body fluids. Conversely, but perhaps less well-recognised, a transient phase of profound anabolism during recovery from illness may substantially lower the plasma urea without any change in renal function.

For all these reasons the plasma creatinine concentration reflects GFR more accurately than the plasma urea. Creatinine is derived from muscle metabolism and is normally cleared by glomerular filtration; under some circumstances (e.g. in nephrotic syndrome) creatinine is secreted into renal tubules and creatinine clearance over-estimates GFR. Consumption of very large quantities (300 g) of cooked meat may double normal plasma creatinine but is a rare source of clinical confusion.

9.

Acid-base Balance

INTRODUCTION

Acid-base has long been the stumbling block of electrolyte therapy: too much physical chemistry, too much physiology, changing concepts and abstract diagnostic parameters have all added to the traditional mystery of acid-base disorders. The three major obstacles have been the use and interpretation of the *pH*, the consequences and the clinical use of the *buffering systems* and the understanding of the *compensatory processes*.

The pH

The acidity of blood (or body fluids) is generally expressed as pH. The normal pH range of 7.36–7.44 corresponds to a hydrogen ion concentration of 44 to 36 nmol/l. A pH outside the range of 6.8–7.8 (corresponding to a H^+ concentration of 158 – 16 nmol/l) is incompatible with life, and values below 7.2 or above 7.5 are potentially dangerous and normally justify intervention, particularly if the derangement is acute.

Acidosis refers to an abnormal physiological process characterised by the gain of acid or loss of base. *Alkalosis* is the reverse. Although a pH < 7.36 (acidaemia) is proof of acidosis and any pH > 7.44 (alkalaemia) leaves no doubt about alkalosis, a pH within the normal range by no means precludes acidosis or alkalosis – or even both of them. This clinically important fact may be due (a) to the action of buffer substances, (b) to secondary, efficient compensating mechanisms, (c) to counterbalancing primary disorders and (d) to any combination thereof.

Buffering Systems

Buffers, by absorbing or donating hydrogen ions according to

86

circumstances, mitigate the pH changes which would otherwise result from the amount of H^+ ions added or withdrawn.

Buffering follows the general equation $HA \rightleftharpoons H^+ + A^-$. Whenever H^+ ions are added, they combine with the buffer base A^- to form the weak acid HA. By this process the H^+ ion is prevented from expressing its activity (which in turn determines the pH of a solution). Conversely, when H^+ ions are wanting, the above reaction is driven to the right, H^+ ions are donated by the weak acid and the change in pH of the buffered solution is less than would be expected from the addition of deficit of H^+ ions. Only weak acids and their salts can act as buffering substances within body fluids.

As a general rule the salts of weak acids with a pK close to the 'normal' or 'physiologic' pH of the body fluids act as the most efficient buffers. (The pK, the negative logarithm of the ionisation constant, is the point at which an acid or an alkali is 50% dissociated; the closer this point is to the plasma pH the better able a weak acid and its salt is to donate or bind hydrogen ions respectively).

Carbonic acid / bicarbonate (pK = 6.1), $H_2PO_4^-/HPO_4^=$ (pK = 6.8), protein buffers (pK = 6.8) and haemoglobin (pK = 6.8) act as the most important buffering systems stabilising the blood pH. Their *in vitro* importance is reflected by the number of mmol of hydrogen ions which would be required to lower the pH of the amount of each buffer contained in a litre of blood from 7.4 to 7.0:

Bicarbonate	18
Phosphate	0.3
Plasma protein	1.7
Haemoglobin	8
	28 mmol H^+

The buffering capacity of bone and the intracellular compartment approximately equals that of the extracellular compartment.

All buffering systems are in contact with a common pool of H^+ ions. The acid base status *in vivo* could therefore be assayed by measuring buffer base and weak acid in any of the above buffering systems. Convenience and tradition, relative importance and readily available measuring techniques have favoured the HCO_3^-/H_2CO_3 system as the major index of acid base changes. With a pK far removed from the pH of extracellular fluid, bicarbonate is hardly an ideal chemical buffer. However, a high molar concentration and the unique properties of bicarbonate/carbonic acid in an open system (CO_2 generated from buffering is excreted via the lungs) render it remarkably efficient in buffering hydrogen ions in biological fluids. The buffering effect of this pair is described by the following equation in which $CO_{2(d)}$ is dissolved CO_2 and the H_2CO_3 concentration is proportional to P_{CO_2} which replaces it in equation (3).

$$CO_{2(d)} + H_2O \rightleftharpoons H_2CO_3 \rightleftharpoons H^+ + HCO_3 \qquad (1)$$

and the interdependence of pH, P_{CO_2} and HCO_3^- is expressed by that stumbling block of ordinary physicians, the Henderson-Hasselbalch equation which reads

$$pH = pK + \log \frac{HCO_3^-}{H_2CO_3}, \text{ or} \qquad (2)$$

$$pH = pK + \log \frac{HCO_3^-}{\alpha P_{CO_2}} \qquad (3)$$

In more detail, the Henderson-Hasselbalch equation is derived as follows:

Since $H_2CO_3 \rightleftharpoons H^+ + HCO_3^-$, at equilibrium the ratio

$$\frac{(H^+)(HCO_3^-)}{(H_2CO_3)}$$

is a constant (K). Solved for (H^+) the equation reads

$$(H^+) = K \cdot \frac{(H_2CO_3)}{(HCO_3^-)}$$

or, taking reciprocals,

$$\frac{1}{(H^+)} = \frac{1}{K} \cdot \frac{(HCO_3^-)}{(H_2CO_3)},$$

and finally, taking logarithms,

$$\log \frac{1}{(H^+)} = \log \frac{1}{K} + \log \frac{(HCO_3^-)}{(H_2CO_3)}$$

or, since

$$pH = \log \frac{1}{(H^+)}$$

and

$$pK = \log \frac{1}{K}$$

$$pH = pK + \log \frac{(HCO_3^-)}{(H_2CO_3)}$$

Apart from water, CO_2 is the main product of metabolism and acts as an acid because it dissolves to form carbonic acid. By regulating the P_{CO_2}, respiration effectively regulates the H_2CO_3 concentration, while the HCO_3^- is regulated by the kidney. Therefore the Henderson-Hasselbalch equation has been parodied, crudely but illustratively, as

$$pH = pK + \log \frac{\text{kidney}}{\text{lungs + respiratory centre}}$$

Although clinical laboratories measure total CO_2 (TCO_2) i.e. the sum of HCO_3^- + dissolved CO_2 gas ($CO_{2(d)}$) + H_2CO_3 and not HCO_3^- alone, the difference between TCO_2 and HCO_3^- is hardly ever greater than 3–4 mmol/l and is of no clinical consequence. $CO_{2(d)}$ and H_2CO_3 are directly proportional to the P_{CO_2} ($0.03 \cdot P_{CO_2}$) and it has therefore to be remembered that abnormal values for P_{CO_2} are to a small extent reflected in the 'bicarbonate' figure traditionally given by clinical laboratories.

The bicarbonate concentration is influenced by bicarbonate gain and loss and, perhaps even more importantly, by losses and accumulation of non-volatile acids in the extracellular space. If non-volatile acids accumulate in the extracellular fluid their hydrogen ions interact with bicarbonate ions; H_2CO_3 is generated and bicarbonate disappears according to the reaction of H^+ + $HCO_3^- \leftrightharpoons H_2CO_3$. H_2CO_3 in biological fluids is quickly split into H_2O and CO_2, which is eliminated by respiration. By these mechanisms the acidity of body fluids is stabilised. Sooner or later, however, the buffering capacity of body fluids (approximately 15 mmol/kg body weight) would be consumed even by the normal daily acid load, unless buffers were regenerated by renal acid excretion and bicarbonate formation.

Compensatory Processes

From the Henderson-Hasselbalch equation it is evident that the pH is determined by the ratio of HCO_3^- : PCO_2 and *vice versa*. By the same token the H^+ ion concentration is defined by the ratio of PCO_2 : HCO_3^- and not by the absolute value of either one alone. This implies that, in terms of pH changes, any primary disturbance of one component (HCO_3^- in primary metabolic; PCO_2 in primary respiratory disorders) can be compensated by appropriate changes in the other: metabolic or respiratory compensation of a primary respiratory or metabolic acidosis or alkalosis. Similarly, two independent respiratory and metabolic disorders will leave the pH of body fluids unchanged provided that the ratio HCO_3^- : PCO_2 (normally $25\,mmol/l : 40\,mmHg$) remains constant.

The chemoreceptors of the respiratory centre normally react quickly to changes in pH of the interstitial fluid of the brain: acidosis increases and alkalosis decreases pulmonary ventilation, but maximal *respiratory compensation* may take 12–24 h to develop, although the first compensatory changes in ventilation are usually apparent within a few hours. This makes respiratory compensation a somewhat sluggish endeavour (though still livelier than metabolic compensatory processes). The delay in response may be due to a slow penetration of hydrogen ions across the blood-brain barrier, the same process that accounts for a delayed fading away of the respiratory response over 12–36 h once the systemic metabolic disorder is corrected. The extent of respiratory compensation depends on the severity of the primary metabolic disturbance and the efficiency of lungs, ventilatory mechanics and respiratory control. However, even with intact pulmonary and respiratory function complete, respiratory compensation of a metabolic disorder is never accomplished and partial compensation (returning the HCO_3^- : PCO_2 ratio *towards* normal) remains the rule.

Renal ('metabolic') compensation of primary respiratory disturbances of acid-base balance is slow and it is based on the kidney's ability to adapt renal acid secretion to the pH and the reabsorption of bicarbonate to the $P\text{co}_2$ of the blood. In respiratory acidosis it becomes apparent within (and not before) 6–18 h in an increased excretion of 'titratable acid', mainly NaH_2PO_4, and reaches its maximum by 5–7 days with an increased distal tubular secretion of NH_3 which combines with the increased amount of H^+ secreted to form NH_4^+.

One of the often perplexing consequences of the sluggishness of *renal* compensation is the phenomenon of seeming 'overcompensation': whenever the primary respiratory disorder rapidly improves hypercapnia and the primary respiratory acidosis improve or disappear, leaving a hang-over of 'posthypercapnic' metabolic alkalosis. Conversely the sluggishness of *respiratory* compensation accounts for the hyperventilation and respiratory alkalosis persisting for hours after the successful correction of a primary metabolic acidosis such as diabetic ketoacidosis.

The time course of the defence of acid-base balance can thus be summarised as follows:

1. extracellular buffering takes place within 10–15 min;
2. additional buffer capacities become available, by diffusion into the intracellular space, during the next 2–4 h;
3. respiratory compensation starts within hours and reaches its maximum within 12–24 h;
4. renal ('metabolic') compensation is not apparent before 6–18 h and takes 5–7 days to reach its maximum.

Symptoms and Signs of Acid-base Disorders

Although the past history and clinical findings often suggest a specific acid-base disorder, few pathognomonic and reliable symptoms and signs are produced by disturbances of acid-base balance.

One of the characteristic signs of *metabolic acidosis* which reflects respiratory compensation is the deep and regular respiration known as Kussmaul's breathing. This sign may be difficult to recognise in mild metabolic acidosis or it may even be completely absent (as seen occasionally in hyperchloraemic acidosis, antidepressant intoxication etc.). With chronic, compensated metabolic acidosis mild hyperventilation is normally sufficient to sustain respiratory compensation. Thus Kussmaul's breathing generally occurs in acute rather than chronic compensated metabolic acidosis. With more severe degrees of acidosis the central nervous system is depressed resulting in headaches, nausea, anorexia, fatigue, confusion, stupor and coma; respiratory depression replaces hyperventilation.

Central nervous manifestations are more frequent and more pronounced with *respiratory acidosis* than with metabolic acidosis because CO_2 readily crosses the blood-brain barrier. In respiratory acidosis, therefore, the pH of the cerebrospinal fluid reliably and quantitatively reflects that of the blood – in contrast to metabolic acidosis, the effect of which on cerebrospinal fluid pH is less marked and more delayed. Increasing fatigue, weakness, abnormal irritability, confusion and delirium, tremor, twitching, papilloedema and eventually coma are the hallmarks of hypercapnia and severe respiratory acidosis.

One of the most important signs of *alkalosis* is increased peripheral and central nervous irritability leading not only to paresthesias and tetany but at times to convulsions. Again, and for the same reasons as discussed before, *respiratory alkalosis* causes more marked symptoms than *metabolic alkalosis*. Acute posthypercapnic metabolic alkalosis is perhaps the only notable exception to this rule.

Compensatory depression of respiration in response to metabolic alkalosis is highly variable. More often than not, compensatory hypoventilation escapes clinical detection and comes as a surprise with the analysis of the acid-base parameters.

INTERPRETATION OF ACID-BASE DATA

The difficulties in interpreting the pH and the parameters describing the state of buffering systems and compensatory mechanisms have led to a search for simplifying concepts and procedures, all of which further practical and quick decisions – sometimes at the cost of a limited understanding of the problems!

Currently three main approaches are adopted to the interpreta-

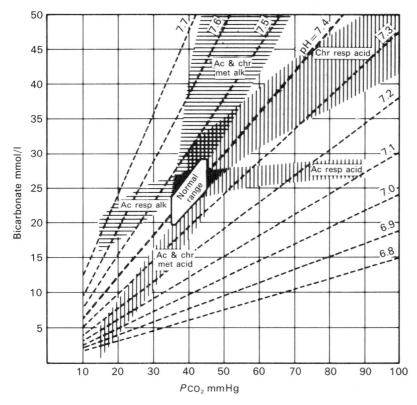

Fig 9.1 The acid-base chart (*in vivo* nomogram for single respiratory or metabolic acid-base disorders) (Originally published in Arbus G.S. (1973), *Canad. Med. Ass. J*; **109**:291.)

tion of acid-base data of which we discuss only the first two in some detail:

1. A graphical approach – the acid-base chart (Fig 9.1).
2. The Siggaard-Andersen terminology and analysis technique.
3. An approach based upon the knowledge of the limits of disturbance and compensation in particular acid-base disorders, using pH, $P\text{CO}_2$ and plasma bicarbonate (total CO_2 respectively) and routine plasma electrolytes as the main laboratory information.

The Acid-base Chart

According to the Henderson-Hasselbalch equation any two of the terms pH, P_{CO_2} or HCO_3^- suffice to describe accurately the acid-base status of a patient. Therefore, two of these terms can be used to define the current situation of a patient by plotting the data on one of the many acid-base charts currently in use. From the position of the point, the nature and extent of the primary acid-base disturbance and the extent of compensatory mechanisms are easily read. Plots of repeated analyses indicate the patient's progress. In addition to its simplicity this method offers the advantage of judging the integrity and completeness of the compensatory mechanisms. The shaded areas indicate the major categories of disturbance and the expected limits of compensation. They also suggest the likely interpretation when a patient's results fall between them.

The 'Siggaard-Andersen' Approach

Instead of using plasma bicarbonate Jorgensen and Astrup have introduced the concept of the *standard bicarbonate*, defined as the bicarbonate concentration found after equilibration of fully oxygenated blood with a P_{CO_2} of 40 mmHg, a measurement which seeks to eliminate *in vitro* the effects of a respiratory component to total bicarbonate. Although the results of this *in vitro* equilibration reflect, they do not necessarily quantitatively represent the *in vivo* situation. Fortunately, in clinical practice the error is small.

Standard bicarbonate offers the advantage of a simple index which reflects the metabolic component of any acid-base disorder. Normal values range from 21 to 25 mmol/l.

Buffer base (BB)

This is defined as the sum of buffer anions of whole blood. It is independent of the P_{CO_2} and reflects the metabolic component of the acid base disorder, just as the standard bicarbonate and the base excess. Normal value 45–50 mmol/l.

Base excess (BE)

The base concentration of whole blood as measured by titration with a strong acid to pH 7.40 at a P_{CO_2} of 40 mmHg and 37° reflects the change in buffer base from its normal value. Obviously it is closely related to the deviation of the standard bicarbonate from its normal value (BE mmol/l = $\triangle$ standard bicarbonate × 1.2). Under normal conditions its value is close to zero. In metabolic acidosis the titration is carried out with strong base and the result is expressed as 'negative BE' (base deficit).

The mathematical relationship between whole blood systems (BB, BE) and the simpler plasma bicarbonate system is complex. Rather than doing mathematical calculations or actual titrations of whole blood, BB and BE as well as standard bicarbonate are read from the Siggaard-Andersen nomogram using two of the three unknowns in the Henderson-Hasselbalch equation, plus the haemoglobin concentration, to derive all the other variables (Fig 9.2).

According to this widely used approach the acid-base situation is split into its respiratory (P_{CO_2}) and metabolic component (standard bicarbonate, BE). With the help of past history, clinical picture and pH it is hardly ever difficult to identify primary and compensatory components. Generally and under steady-state conditions the pH will point to the primary disturbance because, except for chronic respiratory alkalosis, compensatory mechanisms always trail behind the primary component, never fully correcting the pH changes. Unlike the graphic approach, the Siggaard-Andersen technique allows no simple statement of the integrity of the compensating mechanisms.

Thus, a 66-year-old lady with acute-on-chronic asthmatic bronchitis and a P_{CO_2} of 61 mmHg, a standard bicarbonate of 31 mmol/l, a base excess of +8 mmol/l and a pH of 7.37 has a composite acid-base disorder consisting of a respiratory acidosis ($\uparrow P_{CO_2}$) and a metabolic alkalosis (+BE, $\uparrow$ standard bicarbonate). Under steady-state conditions the slightly acid pH indicates a primary respiratory acidosis. To the more experienced observer, however, the abnormally effective metabolic compensation (pH within normal range, standard bicarbonate and BE higher than expected) suggests an additional primary metabolic alkalosis, most probably due to the administration of loop diuretics.

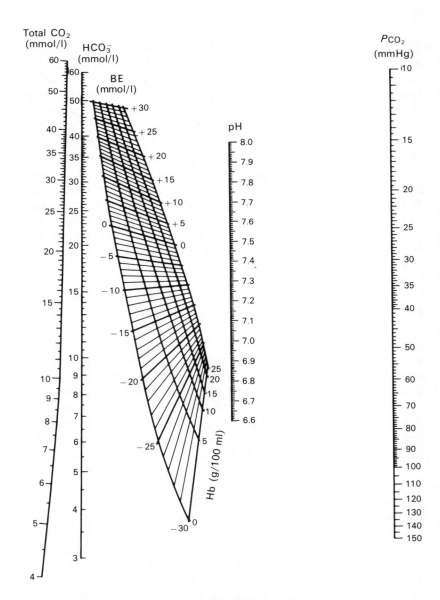

Fig 9.2 Siggaard-Andersen alignment nomogram (*see text*).

An Approach based upon pH, P_{CO_2}, Plasma Bicarbonate (TCO_2) and the Limits of Compensation

This way of analysing acid-base data, which primarily attempts to eliminate the theoretical flaws of the Siggaard-Andersen technique, has recently been outlined by Cohen and Kassirer (*see* references). The approach relies upon an accurate knowledge of how each of the simple disorders of acid-base balance alters the P_{CO_2}, the pH and the plasma bicarbonate (TCO_2), and an equally accurate knowledge of the extent of metabolic and respiratory compensation that can be expected for any given degree and duration of the primary disorders. Actual compensatory processes falling short of or exceeding the expected values may indicate one of the following possibilities:

The patient has not yet had time to, or is not able to mount a normal compensation.

The patient has a second, perhaps a third primary acid-base disturbance superimposed on the already recognised disorder.

The patient has already had time to compensate a seemingly acute primary disorder.

This approach actually is the traditional method of characterising the acid-base status of the blood. Still it is currently not widely used in clinical medicine in European countries and is, therefore, not discussed in more detail in this introductory text. The reader is referred to the references given at the end of this section.

RESPIRATORY ACIDOSIS

Under normal conditions some 15 000 mmol of CO_2 resulting from metabolic processes are excreted daily by the lungs. This balance is sustained by and in turn sustains an arterial P_{CO_2} of 40 mmHg. The processes which impede CO_2 elimination are listed in Table 9.1. The arterial P_{CO_2} increases and only with this hypercapnia is a new equilibrium reached between CO_2 production and CO_2 elimination. Thus an increased P_{CO_2} and respiratory acidosis is the price for CO_2 balance. As a consequence the pH falls and the H^+ ion concentration increases as predicted by

Table 9.1
MAJOR CAUSES OF RESPIRATORY ACIDOSIS

CNS depression	drugs
	lesions/malfunction of respiratory centre*
Neuromuscular disorders	neuropathies
	myopathies
Impaired ventilatory mechanics	
	pneumothorax
	kyphoscoliosis
	flail chest
	scleroderma
Acute/chronic lung disease	acute airway obstruction/asphyxia
	aspiration
	tumour
	laryngeal oedema
	asthma
	chronic obstructive lung disease
	severe pneumonia or pulmonary oedema
Miscellaneous	CO_2 breathing
	cardiorespiratory arrest

* Primary alveolar hypoventilation

the Henderson-Hasselbalch equation and its derivative (equations (2) and (3) p. 88). The hydrogen ions resulting from the reaction

$$CO_{2(d)} + H_2O \rightleftharpoons H_2CO_3 \rightleftharpoons HCO_3^- + H^+$$

are bound by non-bicarbonate buffers, leaving HCO_3^- behind. This process, which never eliminates all H^+ ions produced by hypercapnia, returns the ratio of $HCO_3^- : P_{CO_2}$ and with it the pH *towards*, but not entirely to normal.

After the first 6–12 h *sustained respiratory acidosis* stimulates renal compensatory mechanisms, i.e. an increase in renal excretion of hydrogen ions (mainly buffered by $NH_3 \rightarrow NH_4^+$), a consequent generation of bicarbonate ions and an increased loss of chloride ions (NH_4Cl). As a result, the bicarbonate concentration increases, returning the ratio of $HCO_3^- : P_{CO_2}$ and the pH further *towards*, but not to normal. At the same time, the serum chloride concentration falls causing the typical anion pattern of chronic partially compensated respiratory acidosis.

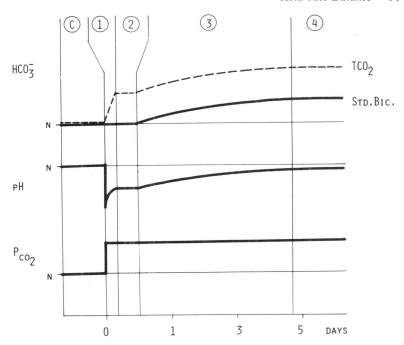

Fig 9.3 Changes in P_{CO_2}, pH, standard bicarbonate and TCO_2 occurring in acute and sustained respiratory acidosis. C = control conditions; 1 = induction of acute hypercapnia, buffering phase; 2 = steady-state acute respiratory acidosis; 3 = increasing renal compensation; 4 = steady-state (maximum) renal compensation in chronic respiratory acidosis.

Although the bicarbonate concentration is higher in chronic than in acute respiratory acidosis because of renal compensatory processes, these mechanisms alone never quite bring the pH back to baseline, even if they often bring it back into the normal range. The stages in buffering and compensation of respiratory acidosis are summarised in Fig 9.3.

RESPIRATORY ALKALOSIS

Respiratory alkalosis as a consequence of acute or chronic alveolar hyperventilation and negative CO_2-balance is due to a number of stimuli to the respiratory centre originating in the

Table 9.2
MAJOR CAUSES OF RESPIRATORY ALKALOSIS

Primary CNS stimulation
functional: anxiety, delirium

	organic brain disease:
	cerebrovascular accidents
	tumour
	infection
	polyneuropathy

drugs	salicylates
	catecholamines
	analeptic drugs

hormones	progesterone
	hyperthyroidism

other	fever
	endotoxaemia/gram-negative sepsis
	liver insufficiency
	pregnancy

Peripheral chemoreceptor stimulation:
hypoxaemia

Intrathoracic receptor stimulation
acute and chronic lung disease
pulmonary embolism
(mild) pulmonary oedema

Acute and chronic mechanical hyperventilation

brain itself, in peripheral chemoreceptors or in intrathoracic receptors (Table 9.2).

Respiratory alkalosis, like respiratory acidosis is generally easily suspected from the patient's past history, clinical findings and overall situation, but it sometimes develops insidiously.

The negative CO_2 balance of alveolar hyperventilation is a transient phenomenon for two reasons: (a) the fall in P_{CO_2} brought about by alveolar hyperventilation limits the rate of pulmonary CO_2 excretion (thus, increased ventilation is gradually offset by its own consequences); (b) the falling P_{CO_2} tends to curb a hyperactive respiratory centre. Both processes eventually lead to a new steady-state in which the rate of CO_2 production equals that of CO_2 excretion by the lungs.

Respiratory alkalosis is characterised by hypocapnia (low P_{CO_2}) and a fall in carbonic acid concentration. The H^+ concentration diminishes and pH increases. In this situation H^+ ions are donated by cellular and extracellular, non-bicarbonate buffers, the bicarbonate concentration falls as the reaction moves to the left.

$$CO_{2(d)} + H_2O \rightleftharpoons H_2CO_3 \rightleftharpoons HCO_3^- + H^+$$

Within the first few hours of respiratory alkalosis the defence of acid-base balance exclusively relies on the extra- and intracellular buffering capacity and it is largely independent of renal compensatory mechanisms. Thus, in *acute* respiratory alkalosis the bicarbonate concentration falls within minutes, but not enough to prevent the pH from increasing. After the first 6–8 h of *sustained* respiratory alkalosis the bicarbonate concentration is lowered beyond the degree expected to result from pure buffering processes. As a compensatory reaction the kidney starts to retain H^+. Respiratory alkalosis causes a mild accumulation of lactic acid; however, the resulting acidosis with 1–2 mmol/l cannot account for the often fully compensating metabolic acidosis found in sustained respiratory alkalosis of more than two weeks' duration. Within the first two weeks of sustained respiratory alkalosis compensation remains incomplete.

The changes in P_{CO_2}, HCO_3^- and pH occurring in acute and sustained respiratory alkalosis are summarised in Fig 9.4.

METABOLIC ACIDOSIS

Primary metabolic acidosis can always be attributed to one of three causative processes (Table 9.3), namely:

1. Increased production or intake of non-volatile acid (e.g. diabetic ketoacidosis, lactic acidosis, salicylate intoxication).
2. Insufficient renal elimination of acids (e.g. acute and chronic renal failure, renal tubular acidosis).

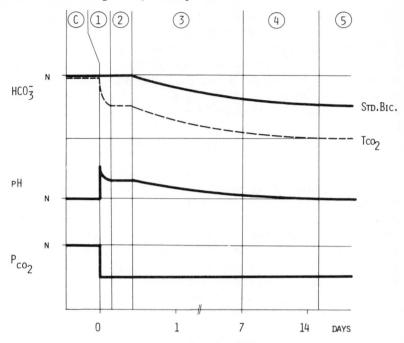

Fig 9.4 Changes in P_{CO_2}, pH, standard bicarbonate and TCO_2 in acute and sustained respiratory alkalosis. C = control conditions; 1 = induction of acute hypocapnia, buffering phase; 2 = steady-state acute respiratory alkalosis; 3 = increasing renal compensation; 4 = steady-state renal compensation in sustained respiratory alkalosis; 5 = full compensation in sustained respiratory alkalosis of more than 2 weeks' duration.

3. Abnormal gastrointestinal or renal loss of bicarbonate (e.g. loss of bile, pancreatic juice or intestinal fluid; renal tubular acidosis).

It has already been pointed out that the hydrogen ions resulting from the acid load are absorbed by extra- and intracellular buffers and that, as the reaction

$$H^+ + HCO_3^- \rightleftharpoons H_2CO_3 \rightleftharpoons H_2O + CO_2$$

moves to the right, hydrogen ions and bicarbonate disappear and an increased amount of CO_2 is eliminated by the lungs. As these

Table 9.3
CAUSES OF PRIMARY METABOLIC ACIDOSIS

Elevated anion gap	*Normal anion gap* *Hyperchloraemic acidosis*
	Hypokalaemia
Renal failure	renal tubular acidosis
Ketoacidosis	diarrhoea
diabetes mellitus	carbonic anhydrase inhibitors
starvation	ureteral diversion
alcohol associated	ureterosigmoidostomy
Lactic acidosis	ileal bladder
Intoxications	*Normokalaemia/hyperkalaemia*
salicylates	chronic adrenal insufficiency
methanol	early renal failure
ethylene glycol	therapeutic use of HCl, arginine-HCl
paraldehyde	or lysine-HCl
	hyperparathyroidism

extra amounts of CO_2 are small compared with the daily production of CO_2, this increased amount of CO_2 does not cause clinically manifest changes in ventilation although if the pH falls respiration is stimulated directly. For similar reasons a primary loss of bicarbonate will shift the above reaction to the left, bicarbonate is generated and a decreased amount of CO_2 is eliminated by the lungs. These buffering reactions and changes in CO_2 excretion (brought about by appropriate changes in alveolar ventilation) occur almost instantaneously and continue as long as the causative abnormality is operative.

In the course of buffering reactions the buffering reserves of the body are gradually consumed and the pH would fall dramatically if the buffer capacity were not regenerated by compensatory mechanisms, i.e. secondary (compensatory) respiratory alkalosis. These mechanisms, become apparent almost immediately. Although, therefore, respiratory compensation is quicker than the renal compensatory process it still may take 12–24 h for maximum response. A second characteristic of respiratory compensation is the fact that, by being proportional to the degree of metabolic alkalosis, it never fully corrects the pH.

The Anion Gap

The sum of unmeasured anions (the so-called *anion gap*, AG) is calculated by subtracting $(HCO_3^-) + (Cl^-)$ from total cations or in first approximation in clinical practice

$$AG = (Na^+) - (HCO_3^-) - (Cl^-)$$

It amounts, normally, to 8–12 mmol/l. With a very few exceptions an increase in AG indicates the accumulation of acid in body fluids. The anions which increase the anion gap in various disorders include sulphate and phosphate and organic anions such as acetoacetate, hydroxybutyrate, lactate, salicylate, oxalate, hippurate, formate and acetate.

The concept of the anion gap has allowed a classification of metabolic acidosis which asks for no more than a simultaneous measurement of sodium, chloride and HCO_3^- (Table 9.3). Although many laboratories no longer routinely measure plasma chloride (which is necessary for the calculation of the anion gap) the concept is useful for understanding and sometimes necessary for diagnosis in the absence of specific measurements.

Of the two most important varieties of high-anion-gap acidosis diabetic ketoacidosis is discussed on p. 135. *Lactic acidosis* (LA) is easily the most acute and severe form of metabolic acidosis.

Under anaerobic conditions glucose is metabolised to lactic acid which dissociates into H^+ and lactate. The plasma concentration of lactate reflects the balance between synthesis (mainly in skeletal muscle, skin and red cells) and oxidation (mainly in liver and kidney). Most disorders which cause lactic acidosis (Table 9.4) inhibit oxidative metabolism either by limiting the oxygen supplied to the tissues or by impairing mitochondrial function. Simultaneously, these processes increase lactic acid production and impair the metabolism of lactic acid to carbon dioxide and water.

The consequences and clinical significance of lactic acid accumulation depend on the plasma concentration and on the patient's initial acid-base status. Minor increases in lactic acid, i.e. concentrations of < 5 mmol/l, do not normally cause a serious metabolic acidosis but superimposed on a pre-existing metabolic or respiratory acidosis even a minor lactic acidosis may result in a life-threatening disorder.

Table 9.4
CAUSES OF LACTIC ACIDOSIS (LA)

1 *Minor* LA (serum lactate < 5 mmol/l)
        Alkalosis
        Exercise
        Alcohol
        Diabetic ketoacidosis
        Carbohydrate infusions
          (mainly non-glucose)
        Catecholamines
        Convulsions

2 *Major* LA (serum lactate > 5 mmol/l)
        Shock
        Hypoxia
        Severe anaemia
        Malignancies
        Biguanides (phenformin)
        Diabetes
        Glycogenoses
        Idiopathic

The *clinical signs* of LA are non-specific. Arteriolar vasodilatation occurs in all forms of severe metabolic acidosis (pH < 7.1) and heart failure may later develop. The clinical diagnosis has therefore to be confirmed by calculation of the anion-gap and, preferably, the direct measurement of the serum lactate (normally 1 mmol/l).

A major LA may develop in a matter of minutes. Lactic acid is a powerful respiratory stimulant and elicits a particularly prompt and energetic respiratory compensation. Often, however, so much acid is produced that severe acidosis results unless the underlying processes are corrected early in the course of the disorder.

Treatment must therefore be aimed primarily at correcting the cause, improving the circulation and tissue perfusion and eliminating potentially causative drugs. In addition, treatment mainly involves the administration of sodium bicarbonate. Severe LA (pH < 7.2) requires massive amounts of alkali and therefore entails substantial danger of fluid overload. Calculation of the alkali need, based on a bicarbonate space of 50% of the body weight (*see* p. 150), provides, at best, a rough approximation of the immediate requirements. Bicarbonate therapy in severe LA should initially aim to keep the plasma bicarbonate above 10 mmol/l. Ancillary therapeutic measures include the adminis-tration of thiamine (3 mg/kg i.m.) and insulin (2–3 u/h i.v.) + glucose as necessary, up to 5 g/h. Dialysis may be neces-sary for removing the causative drugs, reducing ECF volume and even for further correcting the metabolic acidosis.

Whatever the pathogenesis of metabolic acidosis plasma bicar-bonate concentration falls. In order to maintain electroneutrality (total cations = total anions) the resulting deficit in anions is filled by *chloride ions* (so-called hyperchloraemic variety of metabolic acidosis) or by anions, which are not normally measured in the clinical laboratory ('*unmeasured anions*': mainly organic and inorganic anions + anionic proteins; high-anion-gap-variety of metabolic acidosis). The processes of buffering and respiratory compensation occurring in metabolic acidosis are summarised in Fig 9.5, which shows the changes in bicarbonate, pH and $P\text{CO}_2$ expected after an acute acid gain.

METABOLIC ALKALOSIS

Primary metabolic alkalosis is due either to the loss of H^+ from the extracellular space or to a gain of bicarbonate as from the administration of bicarbonate (Table 9.5). The most common forms of metabolic alkalosis respond to the replacement of chloride lost in the development of metabolic alkalosis. Chloride is lost in gastric juice (vomiting and nasogastric suction) and in diarrhoeal fluid in patients with villous adenoma of the colon or congenital chloride-wasting diarrhoea. *Renal* loss of chloride is found during diuretic therapy (except for acetazolamide) and in the course of metabolic compensation of chronic respiratory acidosis (*see* p. 98). In addition to predominant chloride loss, diuretic therapy may induce extracellular volume contraction, another cause of chloride-responsive metabolic alkalosis. Less commonly, metabolic alkalosis occurs *without* chloride loss and, consequently, is chloride-unresponsive e.g. in primary mineralo-corticoid excess and related syndromes.

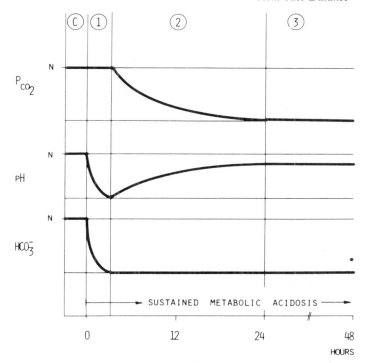

Fig 9.5 Changes in HCO_3^-, pH and P_{CO_2} occurring with acute and sustained metabolic acidosis. C = control conditions; 1 = effect of acid gain/bicarbonate loss + buffering processes, (buffering starts almost instantaneously and continues as long as metabolic acidosis lasts); 2 = increasing respiratory response (hyperventilation); 3 = maximum respiratory compensation (+ continuing buffering processes). * For practical purposes the TCO_2 (total CO_2 content) will be almost the same as the standard bicarbonate.

Normally the kidney compensates for extrarenal losses of acid by retaining hydrogen ions and excreting bicarbonate. There is, however, an important exception to this normal compensation if the process responsible for hydrogen ion loss and metabolic alkalosis also loses chloride and sodium ions. The appropriate renal response to the resulting ECV deficit is sodium retention, but sodium reabsorption in the proximal tubule is limited by a relative deficiency of normally accompanying anion (chloride) and a transport maximum for bicarbonate. A larger load of sodium than normal therefore reaches the distal tubule where,

Table 9.5
CAUSES OF METABOLIC ALKALOSIS

Chloride responsive	*Chloride non-responsive*

Gastrointestinal causes
  vomiting
  nasogastric suction
  villous adenoma diarrhoea
  congenital chloride-
    wasting diarrhoea
Diuretic therapy* and
  contraction alkalosis
  (posthypercapnic alkalosis)
Massive doses of penicillin
  or carbenicillin
	Primary mineralocorticoid excess
	  hyperaldosteronism
	  Cushing's syndrome
	Exogenous 'mineralocorticoids'
	  steroid hormones
	  licorice
	  carbenoxolone
	Bartter's syndrome
	Exogenous alkali load
	Severe potassium deficiency

* Except for acetazolamide

facilitated by the effects of secondary hyperaldosteronism, increased amounts of sodium are reabsorbed in exchange for both potassium and hydrogen ions. Not only is hydrogen ion therefore inappropriately lost by an already alkalotic patient, but a rising plasma bicarbonate is reflected in an increased concentration of bicarbonate in proximal tubular fluid. This results in increasing bicarbonate reabsorption until the maximum ability of the proximal tubule to secrete hydrogen ion is reached. At this point urinary wasting of bicarbonate begins. The whole process, finally, results in the production of a urine with a relatively high pH, a low chloride, an increased potassium and a paradoxically increased sodium concentration.

Elevation of plasma bicarbonate is the hallmark of metabolic alkalosis and results either from bicarbonate administration or from buffering reactions which compensate for H^+ loss. Hydrogen ions are donated by extracellular and intracellular buffers. The reaction of

$$H^+ + HCO_3^- \rightleftharpoons H_2CO_3 \rightleftharpoons H_2O + CO_2$$

is shifted to the left, replacing the missing hydrogen ions and increasing plasma bicarbonate concentration. An equivalent amount of CO_2 disappears and CO_2 excretion by the lungs falls (although in relation to a normal daily excretion of 15–

20 000 mmol of CO_2 this decrease will hardly ever be clinically manifest). By the same token buffering of a primary gain of bicarbonate ions will shift the above reaction to the right and H^+ ions disappear thereby lowering the hydrogen ion concentration and increasing pH. In a second line of defence the $P_{CO_2} : HCO_3^-$ ratio, and with it the hydrogen ion concentration and pH are returned towards normal by increasing the P_{CO_2} through compensatory hypoventilation.

Figure 9.6 summarises the changes in plasma bicarbonate and the processes of buffering and respiratory compensation occur-

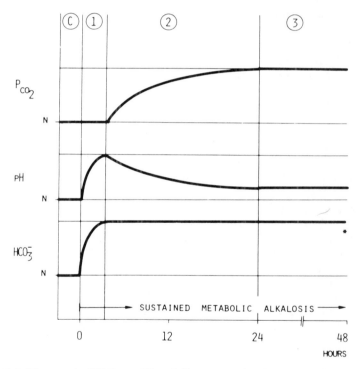

Fig 9.6 Changes in HCO_3^-, pH and P_{CO_2} occurring in acute and sustained metabolic alkalosis. C = control conditions; 1 = effect of acid loss/bicarbonate gain + buffering processes (buffering starts almost instantaneously and continues as long as metabolic alkalosis lasts); 2 = increasing respiratory response (hypoventilation); 3 = maximum respiratory response (+ continuing buffering processes). * For practical purposes the TCO_2 (total CO_2 content) will be almost the same as the standard bicarbonate.

ring in primary metabolic alkalosis. Again, respiratory compensation becomes manifest almost immediately but it may take 12–24 h for maximum response.

MIXED ACID-BASE DISORDERS

Only two of the primary disorders discussed so far cannot occur together: respiratory acidosis and respiratory alkalosis (no patient can have simultaneously a high and a low P_{CO_2}!). With this exception the simple acid-base disorders combine freely with each other producing mixed metabolic or mixed metabolic/respiratory disorders, or even 'triple acid-base disorders', a combination of (primary) metabolic acidosis, metabolic alkalosis and respiratory alkalosis or respiratory acidosis. Mixed respiratory and metabolic acidosis and mixed metabolic acidosis and respiratory alkalosis are the commonest combined disorders.

Further Reading

Cohen J.J., Kassirer J.P. (1982). *Acid-Base*. Boston: Little, Brown & Co.

Kassirer J.P. (1974). Serious acid-base disorders. *N. Engl. J. Med*; **291**:773–6.

Kreisberg R.A. (1980). Lactate homeostasis and lactic acidosis (review). *Ann. Intern. Med*; **92**:227–37.

McCurdy D.K. (1972). Mixed metabolic and respiratory acid-base disturbances: diagnosis and treatment. *Chest*; **62**(suppl.):35S–44S.

Narins R.G., Emmet M. (1980). Simple and mixed acid-base disorders: a practical approach. *Medicine*; **59**:161–87.

Narins R.G., Rudnick M.R., Bastl C. (1980). Lactic acidosis and the elevated anion gap. *Hospital Practice*; **15**:5, 125–35; 6, 91–8.

Seldin D.W., Rector F.C. (1972). The generation and maintenance of metabolic alkalosis. *Kidney Int*; **1**:306–21.

Winters R.W., Engel K., Dell R.B. (1967). *Acid Base Physiology in Medicine. A Self-instruction Program*. Westlake Ohio: London Company.

Appendix

A.

Individual Water and/or Electrolyte Disturbances

SALT AND WATER DEPLETION ('DEHYDRATION')

In clinical practice 'dehydration' usually means salt and water i.e. saline depletion (*see* p. 9).

Diagnosis

The cause, the degree and the relative proportions of salt and water loss must be determined. Neither clinical examination nor biochemical investigation gives the whole answer by itself.

The signs and symptoms of water and of salt and water deficiency are discussed on pp. 11, 12. Postural hypotension is a particularly useful sign of ECF depletion because its significance does not depend on knowledge of an individual's usual blood pressure. Thirst is an early sign of water depletion, but a relatively late sign of isotonic saline depletion.

The plasma sodium concentration is a useful guide to the relative *proportions* of water and salt loss but not to the *extent* of loss. If plasma sodium is normal, the net loss has been isotonic; if it is low, the net loss has been hypertonic in respect to extracellular fluid i.e. saline loss has been replaced by water or, rarely, sodium has been lost in greater proportion than water; if the serum sodium concentration is high, water loss has predominated.

The differential diagnosis of severe dehydration from acute renal failure is discussed in Appendix B (p. 130).

Treatment

1. Weigh the patient to obtain a baseline and weigh daily thereafter.
2. Chart the volume and composition of input and the volume

Table A.1
SUGGESTED OUTLINE OF THE NORMAL APPROACH TO TREATMENT OF SEVERE SALT AND WATER DEPLETION

Plasma sodium	115–145 mmol/l*	> 145 mmol/l
Initial treatment	1 l isotonic (N) saline in 1 h 1 l isotonic (N) saline in 2 h	1 l N/2 saline in 1 h** 1 l N/2 or isotonic saline in 2 h (depending on severity of hyper-natraemia or cerebral symptoms)
Interim treatment	Depending on remaining ECF deficit: 1 l isotonic saline every 4–12 h with a view to correcting the deficit in 48–72 h	Depending on remaining ECF deficit and remaining hypernatraemia: 5% dextrose alternating with iso-tonic saline, 1:2 or 2:1, 1 l every 4–12 h with a view to correcting the deficit in 48–72 h
Continuation (if necessary)	2 l 5% dextrose + 1 l isotonic saline every 24 h + replacement of abnormal fluid loss	

* If $[Na]^+$ < 115 mmol/l and cerebral symptoms are present, start treatment with 200–500 ml 2N saline.
** Although it would seem logical to use 5% dextrose, too rapid a fall in plasma osmolality may result in cerebral oedema.

of output (part of the output may be unmeasurable, e.g. fistulous loss).

3. Roughly estimate the probable overall deficit. It is unlikely that total isotonic saline loss exceeds a third of normal ECF volume, i.e. 4 l in an average adult. Hypotonic losses may be greater because the water loss is taken from a volume three times as large as the ECF volume itself (i.e. ECF + ICF) and is therefore better tolerated. Unless there is continuing abnormal fluid loss, it is reasonable to set a limit on replacement in the first 48 h of 5 l of isotonic saline or 7 l of hypotonic saline or of a combination of 5% dextrose and isotonic saline.

4. A suggested outline of usual treatment of *severe* dehydration designed to avoid too rapid changes in plasma osmolality and plasma volume is given in Table A.1. The precise approach must be determined by clinical and biochemical progress. Convenient oral supplements for use in less serious situations are listed in Table A.2.

Table A.2
ORAL SODIUM SUPPLEMENTS

Preparation	*Table size or content*
Slow-release sodium chloride (slow-sodium, CIBA)	600 mg (10 mmol)
Sodium bicarbonate	600 mg (7 mmol)
Convenient foods	
Chicken noodle soup	200 mmol/l
OXO cubes	4 mmol/g

5. The dangers of excessively large or rapid infusion generally exceed the danger of inadequate or slow replacement. Excessive infusion causes peripheral oedema, pulmonary oedema and – if the plasma sodium concentration is rapidly reduced – intracellular overhydration (including cerebral oedema). It is safer to be a little dry than drowned.

Further Reading
Wendland B.E., Arbus G.S. (1979). Oral fluid therapy: sodium and potassium content and osmolality of some commercial 'clear' soups, juices and beverages. *Can. Med. Ass. J.*; **121**:564–71.

SALINE EXCESS

Diagnosis

Saline overload in excess of about 5 l in an adult of average size causes peripheral oedema. The JVP is raised provided plasma albumin concentration is not low. Pulmonary oedema and effusion are later developments unless left ventricular function is poor, in which case pulmonary congestion or oedema may precede a rise in JVP.

Breathlessness and pulmonary crepitations should be looked for in all patients who may have salt and water overload, especially the elderly.

Treatment

Oedema can normally be controlled by the following sequence of measures:

1. Search for and stop unsuspected sources of sodium intake and sodium-retaining medicines.
2. Give a thiazide diuretic.
3. Substitute or add a loop diuretic (e.g. frusemide). The combination of thiazide and loop diuretics in doses ineffective alone often procures a substantial diuresis.
4. Add spironolactone starting in difficult cases with a near maximal dose of spironolactone (300 mg daily) provided plasma potassium concentration is not high and renal function is not seriously impaired. Spironolactone takes at least 48 h to develop its full effect.
5. Increase frusemide to as large a dose as 2 g daily in exceptional circumstances (or similar loop diuretic appropriately); if unsuccessful give 250 mg or more i.v. because absorption by the oedematous gut wall may be

much reduced; it is useless to give i.m. injections into oedematous tissues. Give the loop diuretic as a once daily dose in this difficult situation to maximise the peak effect. The commonest reason for failure to eliminate oedema is too small a dose of diuretics.

6. If nausea limits the dose of frusemide either substitute another loop diuretic or add a second loop diuretic such as ethacrynic acid (50 mg, 4 x/day).
7. Bed-rest to aid the onset of diuresis.
8. Only if measures 1–6 have failed is it necessary to resort to the unpleasant measure of strict salt restriction.
9. Hypoalbuminaemia: heavy proteinuria should be reduced by treatment with adrenal corticosteroids in patients with corticosteroid-responsive renal disease. A high protein intake is harmful to patients with renal or hepatic insufficiency. If severely hypoalbuminaemic, give an i.v. infusion of salt-poor albumin (75 g) at the same time as a large i.v. dose of diuretic. Although the plasma albumin rise may be small and transitory (especially in nephrotic patients who rapidly lose the infused albumin in their urine) it may be sufficient to trigger diuresis.
10. Haemodialysis (or, as a second-best, peritoneal dialysis) is necessary if a patient with serious saline excess has renal failure. Removal of large volumes of ascitic fluid by paracentesis is dangerous because it causes a sudden fall in plasma volume. Measures such as ultrafiltration and return of ascitic fluid are rarely necessary.
11. If hyponatraemia develops during treatment water intake must be restricted to 500 ml daily.

WATER EXCESS

Diagnosis

Hyponatraemia with reduced plasma osmolality indicates water excess, which may be absolute or relative. Unfortunately, no laboratory test simply differentiates these alternatives but the circumstances of the illness and the simplest signs, including a recent change in body weight, normally allow a correct diagnosis (*see* pp. 11, 12).

Treatment

Normal treatment

When plasma sodium falls below 125 mmol/l water should be restricted to 500 ml daily; plasma sodium should rise by about 3 mmol/l daily.

Emergency treatment

Infusion of hypertonic saline may be necessary to combat deepening coma and fits. Generally 500 ml of 2 N saline suffice to increase the plasma sodium concentration by 5–10 mmol/l in a few hours.

Limitations and Dangers of Treatment

Improvement of symptoms, especially confusion, is slower than the return of plasma sodium concentration to normal in response to treatment.

Intravenous hypertonic saline risks overloading the circulation causing oedema and heart failure. The danger is similar whether 2 N saline or smaller volumes of more concentrated saline are given; the less water is given with the salt the more water will be extracted from ICF into ECF to achieve isotonicity.

The rare patient who without evident cause has a persistent tendency to symptomatic water intoxication can normally be managed satisfactorily by habitual fluid restriction; alternatively health may be maintained by inducing a partial diabetes insipidus-like state with either lithium salts (about 600 mg of lithium corbonate daily) or demeclocycline (about 900 mg daily), both of which interfere with urinary concentrating mechanisms.

Chronic hyponatraemia without symptoms does not require treatment. The patient behaves as if his 'osmostat' were reset, responding normally to deviations below or above his new steady-state.

Intravenous infusion of 5% dextrose or of hypotonic saline

should be used with great care in patients predisposed to abnormal water retention (*see* p. 000).

The hyponatraemia of severe illness and burns, which does not appear to be satisfactorily explained by relative overhydration (*see* p. 29), may sometimes be corrected by the infusion of glucose (600 g daily), insulin (200–400 units daily) and potassium chloride (100–300 mmol daily). It seems likely that the delivery of an intracellular load of potassium promotes an osmotic movement of water into the ICF and possibly also stimulates an exchange of sodium for potassium, both of which outcomes would increase the sodium concentration in ECF.

Further Reading

Schrier R.W. (1978). New treatments for hyponatraemia. *N. Engl. J. Med*; **298**:214–5.

HYPERKALAEMIA

Emergency Treatment

1. *Intravenous 10% calcium gluconate* 10–20 ml or more under ECG control (*see* p. 52). The plasma potassium is not reduced but the membrane effects of hyperkalaemia are antagonised. The effect is immediate and lasts up to an hour; doses can be repeated without loss of therapeutic effect.
2. *Intravenous insulin (10 units) and 50% glucose (50 ml).* Plasma potassium is reduced as potassium moves into cells with glucose. The effect begins within a few minutes and lasts for a few hours.
3. *Intravenous isotonic sodium bicarbonate (1.4%).* 1 l in 2 h is useful in the exceptional patient who is both dehydrated and acutely hyperkalaemic. The effect begins within 15 min and lasts a few hours; potassium moves into cells in exchange for H^+. Most acutely hyperkalaemic patients have acute renal failure and are not suitable for this treatment because their ECF is already overloaded.
4. *Ion exchange resins.* A calcium-cycle resin (calcium poly-

styrene sulphonate – 'Calcium Resonium') avoids the sodium load given in a sodium-cycle resin (sodium poly-styrene sulphonate – 'Resonium A'). 60 g is given in divided doses or 45 g by retention enema, repeated as often as is necessary. The effect is noticeable within 24 h and maintained as long as the resin is taken.

5. If the patient is very catabolic or the cause of hyperkalaemia is not readily reversible *peritoneal or haemodialysis* should be performed as soon as possible.

Long-term Treatment

Dietary restriction of potassium and an ion-exchange resin may be necessary. It is difficult to reduce the potassium intake below 40 mmol daily using conventional foods.

Further Reading
Chamberlain M.J. (1974). Emergency treatment of hyperkalaemia. *Lancet*; i:464–67.

HYPOKALAEMIA

Potassium should not be given i.v. at a rate exceeding 40 mmol/h (3 g of KCl) or in a concentration greater than 40 mmol/l. Ward stock ampoules of potassium must not be used without further dilution. The normal daily requirement is amply covered by about 80 mmol (6 g of KCl). Many potassium depleted patients are also chloride depleted; chloride must be replaced before the potassium deficiency can be corrected (*see* p. 55).

Neither a potassium supplement nor a distal tubular diuretic should normally be given to patients with impaired renal function because of the danger of hyperkalaemia. Potassium supplements are not routinely needed by patients taking diuretics in low dosage as treatment for hypertension. If a potassium supplement proves necessary because of persistent hypokalaemia a dose of at least 2 g (27 mmol) daily will be needed. The precise dose is a matter for trial. Convenient and palatable preparations of potassium are listed in Table A.3. Alternatively a potassium-

Table A.3
CONVENIENT POTASSIUM SUPPLEMENTS

Preparation		*Table size or content*
Soluble effervescent potassium	⎰ 'Kloref'	7 mmol
(mainly as chloride)	⎱ 'Sando K'	12 mmol
Wax-matrix	⎰ 'Slow K'	8 mmol
	⎱ 'Leo K'	8 mmol
Fresh fruit or fruit juice is a more pleasant source of supplementary potassium:		
Fresh orange juice		42 mmol/l
Fresh grapefruit juice		54 mmol/l

sparing diuretic such as amiloride can be added to the diuretic regime or, more effectively in conditions associated with increased aldosterone action, spironolactone given after meals to avoid gastrointestinal irritation.

Combined tablets containing different diuretics or a diuretic and potassium are generally best avoided because individual needs vary considerably. But in the elderly, who need a supplement because of a relatively low potassium intake, a combination tablet (e.g. 'Moduretic' – hydrochlorothiazide 50 mg with amiloride 5 mg) makes for simplicity and is usually satisfactory.

Further Reading

Wendland B.E., Arbus G.S. (1979). Oral fluid therapy: sodium and potassium content and osmolality of some commercial 'clear' soups, juices and beverages. *Can. Med. Ass. J.*; **121**:564–71.

HYPERCALCAEMIA

Severe hypercalcaemia reduces GFR by causing renal vasoconstriction and also impairs both active distal reabsorption of sodium and the sensitivity of the collecting duct to ADH. Hypercalcaemia also causes vomiting. The consequent salt and water deficiency promotes proximal tubular reabsorption of both sodium and calcium, and thus increases hypercalcaemia.

Recommended Procedure

Hypercalcaemia caused by overdosage with vitamin D or by sarcoidosis

1. Stop vitamin D and reduce calcium intake.
2. Rehydrate if necessary with i.v. isotonic saline.
3. If an i.v. infusion is necessary for rehydration add hydrocortisone 50 mg every 6 h. Otherwise start the same dose by mouth or prednisolone 30 mg daily.
4. Reduce prednisolone gradually as soon as calcium falls to normal; a maintenance dose as small as 5 mg daily may suffice and should be continued for three months.

Hypercalcaemia with other cause

Some of the following measures will be needed:

1. *Rehydrate* with i.v. isotonic saline.
2. Give a *loop diuretic* (e.g. frusemide in a dose up to 120 mg every 3 h) replacing water, sodium and potassium losses.
3. *Mithramycin* 25 μg/kg body weight i.v. infusion over 6–8 h, on three or four successive or alternate days. Calcium falls an average of 0.7 mmol/48 h.
4. *Calcitonin* 100 MRC units (25 μg) i.m. or i.v. every 12 h.
5. *Hydrocortisone* 100 mg every 6 h or prednisolone 60 mg daily.
6. *Oral phosphate*. Chronic hypercalcaemia may be satisfactorily controlled with an oral neutral phosphate mixture supplying 1–3 g of elemental phosphorus daily provided it does not cause diarrhoea.
7. *Peritoneal dialysis* (against a calcium-free solution) or haemodialysis.
8. *Treatment of the causative disease* is the only satisfactory long-term treatment.

Further Reading
Anonymous (1980). Management of severe hypercalaemia. *Brit. Med. J.*; **1**:204–5.

HYPOCALCAEMIA

Immediate treatment is only required for tetany or convulsions:

1. Intravenous 10% calcium gluconate 10–20 ml initially or 5% calcium chloride 10–20 ml repeating as necessary to control symptoms.
2. Calciferol or one of its more potent and shorter-acting analogues (*see below*). Repeated measurement of plasma calcium is essential.

Acute Parathyroid Insufficiency

After parathyroidectomy

The problem is more profound after parathyroidectomy for hyperparathyroidism because of an intense healing of osteitis fibrosa which results in hypocalcaemia, hypophosphataemia and hypomagnesaemia. When parathyroid function is damaged at thyroidectomy, the problem is one of acute but usually temporary withdrawal of normal parathormone activity. After parathyroidectomy the following measures should be undertaken:

1. Measure plasma calcium and phosphate daily, magnesium on alternate days for one week; continue at less frequent intervals until the concentrations are satisfactory and stable.
2. 1αOH-cholecalciferol 2 μg every 6 h for 2 days, 2 μg every 12 h for 2 days, then 2 μg daily for 3 weeks. If plasma calcium falls subsequently give either calciferol 1.25 mg or 1αOH-cholecalciferol 1 μg daily if not controlled by calcium lactate gluconate (Sandocal) 1 mmol/kg/day.
3. Calcium lactate gluconate 1 mmol/kg/day and magnesium gluconate 0.2 mmol/kg daily. Continue both for three months, continuing only calcium thereafter if still calciferol-dependent.
4. Relieve painful attacks of tetany with 10% calcium gluconate 10–20 ml i.v. If not relieved by calcium and plasma magnesium concentration is below 0.5 mmol/l give an

Table A.4

CONVENIENT PREPARATIONS OF CALCIUM AND
VITAMIN D

Oral	*Tablet size or content*
Calcium preparations	
Calcium lactate gluconate (Sandocal)	Equivalent to calcium gluconate 4.5 g, i.e. 10 mmol Ca^{++}; 6 mmol Na^+; 4.5 mmol K^+
Calcium and vitamin D preparations (for physiological replacement)	
Calcium and Vitamin D BPC	Calcium sodium lactate 450 mg Calcium phosphate 150 mg Calciferol 12.5 μg (500 units of vitamin D)
Vitamin D preparations (for treatment of hypoparathyroidism or vitamin D resistance)	
Strong calciferol BP	Calciferol 1.25 mg (50 000 units of Vitamin D)
* 1αOH-cholecalciferol ('One Alpha') 1 μg	
* 1,25 dihydroxycholecalciferol, calcitriol ('Rocaltrol')	0.25 μg and 0.5 μg
Injection	
10% calcium gluconate	2.2 mmol calcium/10 ml
Calciferol injection BPC	Calciferol 5 mg (200 000 units vitamin D) in 1 ml depot preparation

* Shorter-acting and therefore easier to control than calciferol.

infusion of magnesium chloride 1 mmol/kg body weight
over 4 h.

5. Long-term treatment with, for example, cholecalciferol
1.25 mg daily or 1αOH-cholecalciferol 1 μg daily will be
needed and must be adjusted according to the plasma
calcium concentration.

After thyroidectomy

When tetany complicates recovery soon after thyroidectomy it can usually be controlled with i.v. calcium gluconate. Recovery of parathyroid function is usually rapid but occasionally long-term treatment with vitamin D is needed as after parathyroidectomy. In such circumstances plasma calcium must be checked every three months for as long as treatment is continued to prevent overdosage or undertreatment.

In other circumstances a supplement of vitamin D with or without calcium is necessary (*see* Table A.4).

HYPER- AND HYPOPHOSPHATAEMIA

Hyperphosphataemia

Hyperphosphataemia is usually the result renal failure. In chronic renal failure hyperphosphataemia can be controlled by measures to reduce intestinal phosphate absorption, such as a high-fibre diet; the use of aluminium hydroxide gel for this purpose, previously the standard treatment, is now less frequently used as a long-term measure because of suspicion that aluminium may cause dementia and osteomalacia associated with regular dialysis.

Hypophosphataemia

An increased intake of milk or a supplement of sodium potassium phosphate is generally sufficient for mild deficiency. Parenteral replacement is necessary for severe deficiency. In uncomplicated asymptomatic hypophosphataemia an initial dosage of 0.08–0.16 mmol/kg body weight (2.5–5.0 mg/kg) should be adequate, the higher dosage being preferred in prolonged and possibly multifactorial hypophosphataemia. Doses are increased by 25–50% in symptomatic patients and decreased to the same extent when significant hypercalcaemia is present. Single doses should not exceed 0.24 mmol/kg (7.5 mg/kg) within 6 h.

Further Reading
Lentz R.D., Brown M.D., Kjellstrand C.M. (1978). Treatment of severe hypophosphataemia. *Ann. Int. Med*; **89**:941–4.

Schneider A.B., Sherwood L.M. (1975). Pathogenesis and management of hypoparathyroidism and other hypocalcemia disorders. *Metabolism*; **24**:871–98.

B.

Clinical Situations

PERIOPERATIVE MANAGEMENT

Electrolyte and fluid therapy has to be tailored to the individual patient, his basic surgical and medical problems, his perioperative condition, his renal, pulmonary and cardiac function and to the results of careful clinical and biochemical assessment over the period of operation.

Fluid and Electrolyte Problems of Anaesthesia, Trauma and Surgery

Anaesthesia, trauma and surgery generate numerous stimuli which alter the regulation of body fluids. Pain, fear, anaesthesia and trauma are potent stimuli to the production and release of ADH. Consequently body fluids become diluted if care is not taken to avoid water intake in excess of this limited ability to excrete water. This tendency persists for 2–4 days after uncomplicated surgery or trauma.

Over the same period the anterior pituitary is stimulated to release ACTH and the plasma cortisol concentration rises up to tenfold. Aldosterone is also increased (for 24–36 h) either in response to ACTH or to stimulation of the renin-angiotensin axis.

This increased mineralocorticoid secretion causes sodium retention and potassium loss, the latter being increased also by glycogen mobilisation and negative nitrogen balance. Thus the early postoperative period is marked by the following:

1. Antidiuresis
2. Retention of sodium
3. Increased potassium loss.

Perioperative Fluid Regimen

Preoperative care

Correct any pre-existing water and electrolyte disorders. Minimise the interval between injury and corrective surgery.

Intraoperative fluid regimen

Replace continuing abnormal losses, losses accumulated during the preoperative fasting period and intraoperative blood loss. With major surgery replace extracellular fluid sequestered during the operative procedure (up to 500 ml of normal saline or Ringer's lactate per hour of operation depending on the procedure and the clinical condition of the patient).

Postoperative fluid regimen

Day of operation ('first postoperative day')
1. Replace urinary and insensible losses as well as the expected minor fluid sequestrations with about 2000 ml of water and 75 mmol NaCl.
2. Replace continuing abnormal fluid losses (nasogastric suction drainage, intestinal secretions etc.) according to volume and their expected (*see* p. 21) or, preferably, measured electrolyte content. Unless the patient is already potassium depleted defer replacement of potassium losses to the next day or the first day when kidney function is known to be adequate.

Second and third postoperative days
1. Increase replacement of 'normal losses' to about 2500 ml of water and 75 mmol Na^+. Replace abnormal losses quantitatively, anticipating the rate of loss on the basis of the amounts of the previous day.
2. Give potassium (60–80 mmol/day) provided renal function is satisfactory.

About the fourth postoperative day most patients with uncomplicated convalescence enter a second postoperative phase: water and sodium handling returns to normal and the daily needs can be safely supplied by 1 l of N saline and 2 l of 5% dextrose. An adequate supply of energy and protein now becomes the first concern. Parenteral nutrition is required early in the postoperative period if there is either a prospect of prolonged postoperative gastrointestinal problems, or other postoperative complications, or the patient was previously in poor nutritional state.

Some authors advocate the administration of larger amounts of sodium and water in the perioperative period. We deliberately prefer a conservative approach modified according to the individual patient's needs, his overall situation and his clinical response.

Further Reading

Bevan D.R. (1978). Intraoperative fluid balance. *Brit. J. Hosp. Med*; **19**:445–53.

Finlayson D.C. (1972). Fluid and electrolyte requirements during anesthesia and surgery. *Anaesth. Analgesia*; **51**:69–74.

Orloff M.J., Hutchin P. (1972). Fluid and electrolyte response to trauma and surgery. In *Clinical Disorders of Fluid and Electrolyte Metabolism* (Maxwell M.H., Kleeman C., eds.) pp. 1063–88. New York: McGraw-Hill.

Shires G.T. (1971). Fluid and electrolyte therapy. *In Manual of Preoperative and Postoperative Care*, 2nd edn. (Kinney J.M., Egdahl R.H., Zuidema G.D., eds.). Philadelphia/London: Saunders.

Shires G.T. (1979). Postoperative, post-traumatic management of fluids. *Bull. N.Y. Acad. Med*; **55**:248–56.

RENAL FAILURE

The sodium, potassium and water disturbances are similar in acute and in terminal chronic renal failure. Acute renal failure is, however, usually reversible while terminal chronic renal failure is the end of the road and only regular dialysis or a renal transplant can give a new lease of life. Chronic renal failure before the preterminal stage offers different problems.

Acute Renal Failure

Diagnosis

Faced with oliguria (urine output less than 400 ml daily) four questions must be asked, although only the differentiation of pre-renal from renal failure is discussed here.

1. Is the cause prerenal (failure of renal perfusion due to factors outside the kidney), renal (intrinsic renal disease) or postrenal (obstruction of renal pelves, ureters or bladder)?
2. If prerenal, is the cause reversible, such as salt and water depletion, acute heart failure or acute peripheral circulatory failure, or is it irreversible, such as renal artery occlusion with infarction of the kidney? If reversible, will correction immediately restore renal function or has the kidney been temporarily damaged?
3. If renal, is the damage reversible, as is the case with 'acute tubular necrosis' (the immediate sequela of renal ischaemia or toxins) or irreversible, such as necrotising glomerulonephritis?
4. If postrenal, the cause should be correctable surgically but does sufficient renal function exist for recovery?

The disturbance of renal function arising from poor perfusion is a spectrum. Differentiation of the extremes of prerenal and renal failure is straightforward. Saline depletion prompts sodium retention: a urinary sodium concentration less than 20 mmol/l in an oliguric patient indicates prerenal failure due to sodium depletion or heart failure. In renal failure the kidney fails to retain the little sodium it filters and the urinary sodium is above 40 mmol/l and may approach that of plasma. In predominant water depletion the urine is concentrated (osmolality usually above 700 mmol/kg; the urine osmolality does not rise so high in response to sodium depletion because the fall in GFR interferes with the countercurrent multiplier system on which urinary concentrating ability depends). In renal failure the small amount of urine formed normally has an osmolality similar to plasma (about 300 mmol/kg, but not infrequently the osmolality is higher (300–400 mmol/kg).

In practice these tests frequently fail to provide a clear separation of prerenal from renal failure. A urine:plasma urea concentration ratio below 10:1 in an oliguric patient indicates established renal damage and with an initial plasma creatinine concentration over 250 μmol/l (>2.8 mg/dl) there is a more than 90% chance of intrinsic renal disease.

An infusion of 500 ml of N saline in 30 min or of 20 g of mannitol is rarely necessary to determine whether the oliguria of sodium and water depletion is immediately reversible. Dehydrated patients increase their rate of urine flow in response; those with acute renal failure do not.

Management of acute renal failure

The major fluid and electrolyte problems of acute renal failure are listed in Table B.1.

Table B.1
THE MAJOR BIOCHEMICAL DISTURBANCES OF ACUTE RENAL FAILURE

1. Fluid overload	salt and water
	water
2. Hyperkalaemia	dietary intake
	endogenous load from catabolism of body protein
3. Acidosis	
4. Retention of drugs and toxic products of protein metabolism	
5. Hypocalcaemia (rarely with transient hypercalcaemia on recovery)	
6. Excessive saline and potassium loss during recovery (rare)	

Fluid overload
Salt and water excess is more readily avoided than treated. Salt intake should be limited in oliguric renal failure (urine output <400 ml/day) to 20 mmol daily and water to the insensible loss – metabolic production (500 ml under normal conditions) + the urine volume of the previous day + any abnormal fluid loss. Dialysis is the only remedy for fluid overload in acute renal failure.

Hyperkalaemia
The emergency treatment of hyperkalaemia is given in Appendix A (*see* p. 119). The dietary potassium should be restricted and no additional potassium should be provided in treatments. At least 4.2 MJ (1000 kcal) should be provided in carbohydrate and fat to minimise protein breakdown and release of intracellular potassium. Peritoneal or haemodialysis may be necessary.

Acidosis
The acidosis of acute renal failure can normally be minimised by restricting protein intake. Treatment with sodium bicarbonate is likely to cause acute pulmonary congestion in patients with renal failure.

Hypocalcaemia
Plasma calcium falls quickly in acute renal failure but requires no treatment. In some cases plasma calcium rises to hypercalcaemic levels during recovery from renal failure.

Excessive sodium, water and potassium loss during recovery
Occasionally the diuresis of salt, water and potassium during recovery from acute renal failure outstrips the cumulative retention and causes deficiency. The greater the degree of overload during acute renal failure (and with good preventive management overload should be avoided) the greater the risk that the ensuing diuresis will exceed the accumulation; rarely, water and electrolyte replacement is necessary during the diuretic recovery phase and must be judged on the clinical findings. Water, sodium and potassium should not be restricted when diuresis is established.

Chronic Renal Failure
(Table B2)

Table B.2
THE MAJOR FLUID AND ELECTROLYTE PROBLEMS OF
CHRONIC RENAL FAILURE

1. Sodium and water	deficiency
	excess
2. Potassium	excess
	deficiency (rare)
3. Acidosis	
4. Calcium	hypocalcaemia (sometimes)
	normocalcaemia with 2° hyperparathyroidism (common)
	hypercalcaemia with autonomous (3°) hyperparathyroidism (rare)
5. Phosphate	hyperphosphataemia

Sodium and water

Patients with chronic renal failure walk a tight-rope between too much and too little salt because they can neither excrete nor retain sodium normally (*see* p. 39). Further, their tolerance changes with time so that the intake appropriate today may not be suitable tomorrow. Excess is easily diagnosed because it causes oedema. Depletion may be difficult to recognise and causes further (but reversible) deterioration of renal function (*see* p. 39).

A therapeutic trial may be necessary to exclude sodium depletion in patients with chronic renal failure who are neither oedematous nor hypertensive; no laboratory test can simply settle the matter. The trial must be conducted in such a way as to minimise the consequences of error. The following is a reasonable approach:

1. Obtain baseline body weight, blood pressure and plasma creatinine and urea; check that there is no oedema and that JVP is normal.
2. Give an oral supplement of 1 g sodium chloride (17 mmol) or 500 mg sodium chloride and 600 mg sodium bicarbonate (7 mmol) if plasma bicarbonate less than 18 mmol/l.
3. Repeat the baseline observations weekly increasing the dose by the same amount as the starting dose each week until either plasma urea and creatinine fall to a new level or peripheral oedema develops, or weight increases by 5 kg, or a raised JVP and/or pulmonary crepitations indicate overload, or blood pressure rises to a level requiring treatment.

Unexplained deterioration of renal function in a patient with previously stable chronic renal failure should be suspected to be the result of saline depletion until proved otherwise.

Potassium

Retention is not normally a problem until the preterminal stage of chronic renal failure. Initially it can be controlled by restriction of intake to below 40 mmol daily but later an ion-exchange resin must be taken regularly. Whether or not sodium-cycle resin is appropriate depends upon whether or not there is associated sodium deficiency. Occasionally, with primary tubular disease, patients with chronic renal failure lose sufficient potassium to require a potassium supplement.

Acidosis

This is hardly ever mainly responsible for the symptoms of chronic renal failure. Complete correction would generally require an amount of sodium bicarbonate greater than could be excreted. The total plasma calcium concentration is often low but the ionised calcium (increased in acidosis) is usually normal. Correction of acidosis reduces the ionised calcium and entails a risk of provoking convulsions.

Calcium

If the plasma calcium is low the patient should be treated cautiously with vitamin D; a large daily dose of calciferol (1.25 mg) or a physiological dose of analogues which are not dependent upon their hydroxylation in the kidney (1 μg of 1αOH-cholecalciferol or 0.25 μg of 1,25-dihydroxycholecalciferol) is necessary to correct hypocalcaemia in chronic renal failure. Overtreatment is dangerous because hypercalcaemia eventually irreversibly damages the kidney. These large doses of vitamin D should never be given without checking plasma calcium frequently.

Total parathyroidectomy is necessary in the rare patient whose parathyroid overcompensates and causes hypercalcaemia ('tertiary hyperparathyroidism').

Phosphate

Severe hyperphosphataemia should be prevented in chronic renal failure. Administration of oral aluminium hydroxide gel to bind phosphate in the gut was the standard treatment but aluminium may cause dementia and osteomalacia in patients on regular dialysis. The use of phytate or a high-fibre diet is probably preferable.

LIVER FAILURE

Pathophysiology

The two problems of immediate relevance to body fluids are salt and water retention triggered by hypoalbuminaemia and hypokalaemia; both the sodium retention and hypokalaemia are logically remedied by blocking secondary hyperaldosteronism.

Treatment

Salt and water retention

Oedema and ascites can normally be controlled with diuretics, especially the combination of a thiazide, a loop diuretic and a large dose of spironolactone (*see* p. 116). The commonest cause of failure to control oedema and ascites is too small a dose of diuretics. Salt should not be added to food but a strict low-salt (20 mmol) diet is only occasionally necessary.

Hypokalaemia

Hypokalaemia in association with chronic liver disease is attributable to secondary hyperaldosteronism, large doses of loop diuretics and poor intake. Hypokalaemia predisposes to liver coma. A large dose of spironolactone is needed; occasionally a potassium supplement is also required.

UNCONTROLLED DIABETES MELLITUS

Pathogenesis

The patient is saline depleted because of vomiting and the osmotic diuresis caused by heavy glycosuria and is usually (but not invariably) ketoacidotic as a result of insufficient insulin. Potassium depletion is masked initially by a normal or even high plasma potassium concentration. Intracellular potassium is exchanged for hydrogen ion as acidosis develops but a reverse shift occurs when the acidosis is corrected.

Too rapid correction of a water deficit especially in hyperosmolar patients may cause cerebral oedema and too rapid replacement of saline may cause pulmonary oedema. The biochemical disturbances of uncontrolled diabetes have usually taken several days to develop and are most safely corrected over a day or two, especially in the elderly and in children.

Biochemical Investigations

Frequent biochemical tests are essential to guide optimum treatment:

1. Blood glucose 2-hourly until glucose is <15 mmol/l.
2. Plasma potassium 2-hourly until glucose controlled, then daily for up to 1 week.
3. Plasma sodium and urea or creatinine 4-hourly until glucose controlled.
4. Arterial pH, P_{CO_2} and standard bicarbonate 2-hourly until pH >7.2.

Treatment

General management

Introduce CVP line.
Aspirate stomach if patient is drowsy to prevent aspiration of vomit.
Catheterise bladder and leave indwelling catheter until consciousness regained.
Chart all intake and output.

Fluid and electrolyte replacement

A suggested scheme for ECF and potassium replenishment is given in Tables B.3 and B.4. Modifications will be needed in unusual circumstances; for example, the more acute the disturbance the smaller the ECF volume loss may be and the suggested replacement volumes should be reduced. Body size must also be

Table B.3
SCHEME FOR FLUID REPLACEMENT IN AN ADULT WITH
UNCONTROLLED DIABETES

Duration of infusion of each l	Initial plasma sodium <145 mmol/l	>145 mmol/l
1 h	*N saline	N/2 saline
2 h	*N saline	N/2 saline
3 h	N saline	N/2 saline until [Na] <145 mmol/l then N saline
4–6 h unitl blood glucose <15 mmol/l	N saline	
8 h	5% dextrose until diabetes controlled and water deficit corrected	

* Consider replacing with isotonic (1.4%) sodium bicarbonate if severely
acidotic (pH < 7.0) and plasma potassium > 4 mmol/l; it is very rarely
necessary to use bicarbonate at all and many physicians avoid it altogether
because of the risk of inducing hypokalaemia during rapid correction of
acidosis.

Note: The rate of repletion will have to be slowed if the CVP rises or if there are
signs of pulmonary congestion or if urine output does not increase as expected.
The volume of repletion must be considered in the light of all the clinical
circumstances including body size (*see text*).

Table B.4
SCHEME FOR POTASSIUM REPLACEMENT IN AN ADULT
WITH UNCONTROLLED DIABETES

	Initial plasma potassium low	normal	high
First hour	40 mmol	27 mmol	nil
Second hour	27 mmol	13 mmol	13 mmol
Subsequent hours for duration of maximum insulin dose		13 mmol	
Subsequent days if i.v. infusion needed when on reduced insulin dose	40 mmol/day i.v. + 27 mmol/day oral in addition to diet, provided renal function is adequate		

The rate of repletion will have to be reduced if renal function is poor and fails to
improve. Rarely a faster rate of repletion is required. A good case can be made
for giving half the oral potassium replacement as phosphate if renal function is
normal and plasma phosphate is low. 40 mmol = 3g KCl.

taken into account together with signs of ECF depletion in deciding the appropriate repletion volume.

Insulin

Do not give any insulin until plasma potassium is known to be at least 4 mmol/l or potassium replacement has commenced.

Use highly purified soluble insulin:

Give an initial i.v. bolus of 20 u followed by continuous i.v. infusion with pump 5 u/h *or* 20 u i.m. (or 10 u i.v. and 10 u i.m.) followed by 5 u i.m./h until plasma glucose <15 mmol/l, then s.c. insulin every 4–8 h according to need.

In the rare instance when plasma glucose is not falling within 2 h of starting treatment a second bolus insulin dose of at least 20 u should be given i.v. and more if necessary.

Further Reading

Reith S. (1977). Management of diabetic coma. In *Clinical Medicine and Therapeutics I* (Richards P., Mather H., eds.) pp. 154–9 Oxford: Blackwell.

SEVERE DIARRHOEA

Acute Diarrhoea

Pathophysiology

Diarrhoeal fluid usually has about two-thirds of the sodium concentration and five times the potassium concentration of plasma. The water and electrolyte losses are increased if the patient is also vomiting (*see* p. 21).

Enterotoxic bacteria cause diarrhoea by producing a protein which binds tightly to intestinal epithelial cells and increases their adenyl cyclase activity and their concentration of adenosine 3′, 5′-cyclic monophosphate (cAMP). Accumulation of cAMP results in increased net secretion of salt and water by intestinal epithelial cells both by inhibiting saline absorption and stimulating the secretion of sodium bicarbonate. Glucose entry into cells is, however, unaffected and the glucose-carrier permits the entry of one molecule of sodium with each glucose molecule, a point of cardinal therapeutic importance.

Treatment

1. Inhibit vomiting with i.m. prochlorperazine or chlorpromazine.
2. Most patients soon stop vomiting and are safely, effectively and cheaply treated orally with solution of N/2 saline (75 mmol/l) and glucose (75 mmol/l) with potassium added as necessary (usually 27 mmol/l), or sodium chloride and dextrose compound powder BPC dissolved in water to give a solution containing per litre sodium 35 mmol, potassium 20 mmol, chloride 37 mmol, bicarbonate 18 mmol and dextrose 200 mmol.
3. If vomiting prevents oral treatment give i.v. N saline alternating with 5% dextrose in the ratio of 1:1 or 1:2 according to plasma Na^+ with potassium added as necessary, usually 27 mmol/l, at a rate sufficient to replace continuing losses and to correct the initial deficit.

Chronic Diarrhoea

Pathophysiology

Potassium depletion dominates the biochemical disturbance of chronic diarrhoea. Water loss is normally corrected spontaneously through thirst.

Because the intestinal transit time is slower than in acute diarrhoea, the sodium concentration of the faecal fluid is also lower, provided the colon and rectum are not extensively diseased. Sodium conservation is aided in both kidney and colon by secondary hyperaldosteronism but potassium loss is correspondingly increased; paradoxically therefore the less intrinsically diseased the colon and the more effective its ability to reabsorb sodium in exchange for potassium the larger the potassium loss, which may explain why purgative abuse is such as powerful cause of diarrhoea-mediated hypokalaemia.

Treatment

Potassium chloride supplements (in soluble rather than slow-release preparations) are needed in addition to treatment of the underlying disease. In chronic diarrhoea with substantial bicarbonate loss the potassium replacement is better given as bicarbonate.

Further Reading

Anonymous (1975). Oral glucose-electrolyte therapy for acute diarrhoea. *Lancet*; **i**:79–80.

Phillips S.F. (1972). Diarrhoea: a current view of the pathophysiology. *Gastroenterology*; **63**:495–518.

Pierce N.F., Sack R.B., Mitra R.C. *et al*. (1969). Replacement of water and electrolyte losses in cholera by an oral glucose-electrolyte solution. *Ann. Intern. Med*; **70**:1173–81.

PYLORIC STENOSIS

Pathophysiology

Pyloric stenosis results in sodium and water depletion, potassium depletion and metabolic alkalosis on account of:

1. The loss in vomit of water, sodium, chloride and H^+ (potassium loss is small but intake is prevented);
2. Renal potassium loss due to secondary hyperaldosteronism and to a limitation of proximal tubular reabsorption of sodium by a relative unavailability of chloride, which results in an increased distal reabsorption of sodium in exchange for potassium and H^+;
3. Continuing renal H^+ loss because of both secondary hyperaldosteronism and the effects of chloride deficiency as in (2) above.

Treatment

General measures

Aspiration of gastric contents through a nasogastric tube relieves vomiting and often restores gastric drainage by removing solid residues and allowing oedema to subside.

Temporary cessation of oral feeding, intermittent gastric aspiration and appropriate treatment of a peptic ulcer, if associated inflammation is the cause of pyloric stenosis, may be sufficient treatment. In most cases a degree of fixed obstruction remains caused by fibrous scarring or tumour in which case surgery is required.

Sodium, chloride and water replacement

The sodium concentration of gastric juice is about 75 mmol/l: the sodium and water loss can therefore satisfactorily be replaced by alternating N saline with 5% dextrose to a total initially of 3 or 4 l daily. This fluid replacement provides a chloride concentration also of 75 mmol/l but the loss in gastric juice is nearer 100 mmol/l; additional chloride must therefore be given with potassium.

Potassium replacement

Body potassium cannot be adequately replenished until the renal potassium wasting is stopped. Replacement of sodium and water reduces renal potassium loss by correcting secondary hyperaldosteronism but chloride must also be provided before distal tubular sodium exchange for potassium and H^+ is reduced to normal. As long as the patient remains hypokalaemic 40 mmol (3 g) of potassium chloride chould be added to each litre of intravenous fluid.

Correction of alkalosis

Not until secondary hyperaldosteronism and chloride deficiency have both been corrected can the alkalosis be corrected; correction of potassium deficiency enables H^+ to be released from ICF in which it had substituted for potassium and makes more

potassium available for the distal tubular exchange, thus sparing
H^+. Diminished tubular secretion of hydrogen ions results in
reduced bicarbonate reabsorption; increased urinary bicarbonate
excretion corrects the alkalosis.

ADRENAL INSUFFICIENCY

Acute Adrenal Insufficiency (Addisonian Crisis)

Recommended procedure

1. Intravenous plasma to restore blood pressure plus intravenous hydrocortisone 200 mg *or*
2. 1 l isotonic saline (preferably containing 5% dextrose to
   correct hypoglycaemia) + 200 mg of hydrocortisone i.v. in
   1 h.
3. 1 l isotonic saline in 2 h
4. 1 l isotonic saline + 100–200 mg hydrocortisone in 6 h (continue at the same or reduced rate for 24 h according to
   clinical signs of adequacy of ECF replacement.
5. Hydrocortisone 20–50 mg oral or i.v. in every 6 h for next
   24 h.

Chronic Adrenal Insufficiency

1. Cortisone 25 mg in morning and 12.5 mg in evening or
   hydrocortisone 20 mg in morning and 10 mg in evening;
   these doses should be increased four-fold in the event of
   intercurrent illness, injury or operation.
2. Fludrocortisone 100 µg daily (more or less as necessary to
   provide mineralocorticoid supplement).

Further Reading
Hall R., Anderson J., Smart G.A., Besser M. (1975). *Fundamentals of
Clinical Endocrinology*, 2nd edn., pp. 155. London: Pitman Medical.

DIABETES INSIPIDUS

Differentiation of Pituitary from Renal Diabetes Insipidus

The clinical history and presence or absence of other disease provide important clues. The renal response to antidiuretic hormone, now available in the synthetic preparation desmopressin (1-deamino, 8-D-arginine vasopressin, DDAVP) provides a simple but not always discriminating test; measurement of plasma arginine-vasopressin (AVP) is better (low or absent in pituitary and high in renal diabetes insipidus) but not yet generally available.

A convenient procedure for a desmopressin test is as follows:

1. Warn the patient not to drink excessively for 24 h to avoid headache from intracerebral overhydration.
2. Ensure that urine has recently been passed.
3. Give 40 μg desmopressin by i.n. instillation.
4. Measure the osmolality of each specimen of urine passed during the next 9 h; often only one or two specimens are passed.
5. An osmolality above 700 mmol/kg is expected if the kidneys are normal but may be little over 300 mmol/kg if a high fluid intake is habitual. The urine osmolality of patients with polyuria due to renal diabetes insipidus does not rise much above 300 mmol/kg in this test.
6. In case of doubt repeat the test with 20 μg desmopressin i.m. lest intranasal instillation was improperly given or intranasal pathology has impaired absorption.

Differentiation of Pituitary or Renal Diabetes Insipidus from Compulsive Water Drinking

The clinical, social and psychiatric history is more important than any laboratory test; pregnancy should be excluded.

The differential diagnosis is especially difficult because hypothalamic-pituitary lesions variably affect ADH secretion and thirst. Some patients have polyuria as a result of increased thirst while ADH secretion is adequate. The patients most at risk are those with both ADH deficiency and decreased thirst.

A desmopressin test may give an equivocal result because the urine concentrating ability is impaired in all individuals who habitually drink large volumes of fluid. Even measurement of ADH may fail to differentiate between partial hypothalamic diabetes insipidus and primary polydipsia unless the plasma AVP concentration is measured under defined conditions of dehydration or infusion of hypertonic saline and is interpreted in the context of concurrent plasma and urinary osmolalities.

The response of body weight, plasma osmolality, urine osmolality and urine volume to 24 h of fluid deprivation gives most information. The initial plasma osmolality is usually low-normal (around 280 mmol/kg) in a compulsive water-drinker and high-normal (normal 300 mmol/kg) in a patient with diabetes insipidus. The plasma sodium concentration will be 135–140 mmol/l in the former and 140–145 mmol/l in the latter. Unfortunately there is too much overlap for these to be reliable differentiators.

In a compulsive water-drinker body weight hardly falls, plasma osmolality rises little, urine osmolality rises and urine volume falls in response to fluid deprivation. By contrast, in diabetes insipidus body weight falls, plasma osmolality rises above the normal range, urine osmolality rises little and urine volume does not greatly diminish.

Pituitary Diabetes Insipidus

Acute

Acute diabetes insipidus after head injury or neurosurgery is usually temporary and only requires careful attention to fluid balance.

Chronic

Mild cases can often be satisfactorily controlled with a thiazide diuretic (*see* p. 27) or by chlorpropamide (*see* p. 31). Desmopressin, a synthetic analogue of ADH, can be given intranasally (40 μg) or by intramuscular injection (2 μg). A sublingual preparation may soon be available.

Renal Diabetes Insipidus

The kidney is insensitive to ADH. Urine flow may be reduced by treatment with a diuretic (*see above*).

Further Reading

Monson J.P., Richards P. (1978). Desmopressin urine concentration test. *Brit. Med. J*; **1**:24 and 105.

Stern P., Valtin H. (1981). Verney was right, but . . . (the differential diagnosis of diabetes insipidus). *N. Engl. J. Med*; **302**:1581–2.

Stuart C.A., Neelon F.A., Lebovitz H.E. (1980). Disordered control of thirst in hypothalamic-pituitary sarcoidosis. *N. Engl. J. Med*; **303**:1078–81.

Vaamonde C., Presser J.I., Clapp W. (1974). Effect of high fluid intake on the renal concentrating mechanism of normal man. *J. Appl. Physiol*; **36**:434–9.

ELECTROLYTE INTERACTIONS IN THE THERAPEUTIC USE OF LITHIUM SALTS

The margin between the therapeutic plasma concentration of lithium (0.7–1.3 mmol/l) and the toxic (2 mmol/l) is narrow. Sodium and, to a lesser extent, potassium depletion results in an increased plasma lithium concentration, thus increasing the chance of toxic effects.

The major potential electrolyte pitfalls associated with lithium treatment are:

1. *Initial lithium and water retention* causing weight gain, especially if given with a monoamine-oxidase inhibitor. The danger is that a diuretic will be given and will increase plasma lithium if sodium diuresis exceeds lithium diuresis.

2. *The use of a diuretic for coincidental illness* e.g. hypertension. A diuretic can be given safely but the dose of lithium needs to be reduced initially and its plasma concentration must be checked until a new steady state is achieved.

3. *Polyuria and polydipsia as a result of lithium-induced renal diabetes insipidus.* These symptoms occur in about 10% of

patients, and are usually reversible; lithium should normally be stopped.

Treatment of Lithium Overdosage

Forced diuresis is a simple and satisfactory treatment. The tendency to excrete very dilute urine as a result of insensitivity to ADH makes it appropriate to use, for example, isotonic sodium chloride alternating or in the ratio of 1:3 with 5% dextrose; both Na and K depletion must be avoided. Peritoneal and haemodialysis are safer alternatives.

Further Reading

Anonymous. (1977). Adverse effects of lithium treatment. *Brit. Med. J*; iii:346.

Forrest J.A.H. (1975). Forced diuresis for lithium intoxication. *Postgrad. Med. J*; 51:189–91.

BURNS

This short discussion is limited to the *fluid* problems of the burned patient. General surgical problems of burns are not considered. For more details the reader is referred to additional reading listed at the end of the section.

Pathophysiology

Although a precipitous fall in cardiac output has been reported to precede any measurable change in plasma and blood volume, and although the survival of the burned patient is influenced by a number of important additional factors, optimum fluid therapy is essential.

Plasma volume is initially depleted by leakage from damaged capillaries. Fluid accumulates in the interstitial space at a rate of approximately 2 ml/kg% of burn in the first 12–18 h with a 40% burn. Capillary integrity recovers in the second 24 h period after a burn and plasma volume may even increase as some of the interstitial oedema fluid returns to the circulation.

The evaporative water loss through the burned skin from the first to the fourth day after injury is several times normal depending on the area and depth of burn. As the crust dries over second degree burns evaporative water loss diminishes but remains greater than normal until the burn heals or is grafted. This persisting surface water loss poses a dual problem of maintaining water balance and a continuing drain on energy stores because energy is used in the process of evaporation.

The increase in metabolic rate associated with burns greatly exceeds other types of injury. The daily energy requirements are increased by about 4.2 MJ (1000 kcal) for each 10% burn area. Thus the daily expenditure of a moderate to severely burned patient may well amount to 16.8–25.2 MJ (4000–6000 kcal), while the protein requirement is calculated as 70 g + 1 g per % burn. Modern techniques of parenteral feeding enable these requirements to be met even when the enteral route fails.

Fluid Therapy

Whereas most approaches in the past have advocated the simultaneous use of colloids and crystalloids (Alternative 1, Table B.5) colloids rapidly pass from the vascular bed into the interstitial compartment in the first 24 h after burn and therefore they exert

Table B.5
FLUID RESUSCITATION THERAPY DURING THE EARLY POSTBURN PERIOD (FIRST 48 h AFTER BURN)

	Alternative 1	Alternative 2
First 24 hours		
Colloid[1]	0.5 ml/kg/% burn[3]	nil
Electrolyte[2]	1.5 ml/kg/% burn	4 ml/kg/% burn
5% or 10% dextrose	2000 ml	nil
Second 24 hours		
Colloid[1]	0.25 ml/kg/% burn	0–2000 ml
Electrolyte[2]	0.75 ml/kg/% burn	nil
5% or 10% dextrose	2000 ml	2–4000 ml

[1] Plasma, human serum albumin or dextran
[2] 0.9% saline or Ringer lactate
[3] To be assessed on the basis of the 'rule of nine's'; each lower extremity, the anterior and posterior trunk are allocated 18% of the body surface (each), each upper extremity and the head are considered as 9% (each), and the remaining 1% is allocated to the neck and/or perineum.

no more than a transient oncotic effect. An alternative approach (Alternative 2, Table B.5) reserves colloids for the second 24 h period when a restored capillary integrity will allow the build-up of a colloid osmotic pressure gradient between the vascular and the interstitial compartment. Both these fluid resuscitation plans serve as a rough guide to be modified according to the patient's individual circumstances. In particular, 'burn shock' (which is the result of ECF loss) must be managed with regard to pulse, blood pressure, peripheral perfusion and urine output.

The loss of plasma volume is most rapid within the first 8 h after injury and half of the fluid prescribed for the first day should be given during the first 8 h.

Metabolic acidosis (lactic acidosis and/or renal acidosis) commonly complicates major burns and is treated by giving part of the sodium requirement as bicarbonate instead of chloride.

Potassium is lost from burned tissues, initially causing hyperkalaemia and later hypokalaemia (by the second post-burn week). Potassium supplements should be given as soon as hypovolaemia has been corrected and urinary output and renal function have been restored.

Thermal injury may destroy a significant fraction of the red blood cell mass. In the early post-burn period one-third to one-quarter of the colloid replacement is given as whole blood.

The fluid problems of minor burns (up to 20% of body surface) can usually be corrected by the oral route. An oral salt solution containing 2.5 g NaCl + 2.5 g NaHCO$_3$ per litre of water, chilled, sweetened and flavoured to the patient's tast is usually well tolerated and may greatly simplify fluid replacement therapy.

Further Reading

Baxter C.R. (1974). Fluid volume and electrolyte changes in the early post-burn period. *Clin. Plast. Surg*; **1**:693–709.

Baxter C.R. (1978). Problems and complications of burn shock resuscitation. *Surg. Clin. N.Amer*; **58**:1313–22.

Hinton P., Allison S.P., Littlejohn S., Lloyd J. (1973). Electrolyte changes after burn injury and effect of treatment. *Lancet*; **ii**:218–21.

Moncrief J.A. (1973). Medical progress: burns. *N.Engl. J. Med*; **288**:444–54.

Muir I.F.K., Barclay T.L. (1962). *Burns and Their Treatment*. London: Lloyd-Luke.

Pruitt B.A. (1978). Fluid and electrolyte replacement in the burned patient. *Surg. Clin. N.Amer*; **58**:1291–312.

TREATMENT OF ACID-BASE DISORDERS

Respiratory Acidosis

Treatment of acute and chronic respiratory acidosis primarily aims at reducing the P_{CO_2}. In acute respiratory acidosis this goal can be pursued without hesitation. In contrast, in *chronic* respiratory acidosis, posthypercapnic metabolic alkalosis and its clinical consequences (arterial hypotension, cardias arrythmias, confusion, delirium and seizures) limit the extent to which the P_{CO_2} is allowed to fall. The administration of chloride ions and acetazolamine under these conditions hastens the reduction of the compensatory metabolic alkalosis. Whether acetazolamide is a useful adjunct in the treatment of a patient with chronic respiratory failure who is not mechanically ventilated remains a matter of debate. Acetazolamide diminishes the renal compensation of chronic respiratory acidosis. This enforced acidosis may stimulate the respiratory effort and lower the P_{CO_2}. In practice the benefits are uncertain. The use of TRIS-buffer (tris-hydroxy-methylamino-methane), the only buffer available for clinical use which is able to buffer carbonic acid (except for bicarbonate!), should not be attempted without mechanical control of respiration and then only with expert supervision.

Adequate oxygenation remains one of the most important goals in treating respiratory acidosis.

Respiratory Alkalosis

The treatment of primary respiratory alkalosis is generally directed at the cause. This may be accomplished by psychotherapeutic measures, by pharmacological sedation of the hyperactive respiratory centre, by improving or eliminating hypoxic stimuli or, if necessary, by rebreathing methods – breathing gas mixtures with an increased P_{CO_2} (5 vol%).

Metabolic Acidosis

The treatment of metabolic acidosis aims at the underlying disorder and at restoring the buffer capacity by administering base. Bicarbonate, the base of the most important extracellular buffering system, is most suitable. Sodium acetate and sodium lactate have to be metabolised to $NaHCO_3$ and offer no advantage in buffering effect over bicarbonate. The same holds for TRIS whose side effects (respiratory depression, hypoglycaemia, hypokalaemia and local venous irritation related to its alkalinity) make it a rather undesirable substance. It has been claimed, but not proved, that TRIS will cause less extracellular volume expansion than equivalent amounts of sodium bicarbonate. In view of an apparently better penetration of TRIS into the intracellular space, this claim may well be true. Whether it outweighs the undesirable side effects, is still a matter of debate.

The intensity of treatment and the amounts of buffering substances to be administered very much depend on the underlying disease and on the degree of metabolic acidosis. It is usually not desirable to achieve a full correction of the bicarbonate deficit rapidly. Patients continue to hyperventilate for hours after the acute correction of metabolic acidosis, producing respiratory alkalosis because of the delayed response of the respiratory centre.

Approximate calculations of the bicarbonate deficit which assume a 'bicarbonate space' of 50% of body weight (bicarbonate deficit = $0.5 \times BW \times$ the deviation of bicarbonate from normal) serve as a rough and strictly momentary estimate of the buffer deficit and buffer requirement, rather than as a quantitative prescription to be fulfilled within the next 24 h. We prefer a step-by-step approach, in which each step depends on the extent of the disorder and the success of previous therapeutic measures. Generally 50 mmol $NaHCO_3$ per h is a reasonable rate at which to administer base. However, if the endogenous production of acid continues (as in lactic or ketolactic acidosis) this rate may prove utterly inadequate. The enormous amounts of bicarbonate required in some of these patients (up to 100 mmol per hour, several hundred mmol of $NaHCO_3$ within a few hours) soon cause serious problems of extracellular volume excess and circulatory overload. In this situation, the use of 1-molar sodium bicarbonate, more often than not, only replaces volume problems by the problems of hypernatraemia and hyperosmolality. Peritoneal and haemodialysis may offer the only solution.

In acute and chronic renal failure the risk of extracellular volume overload has to be carefully weighed against the advantages of a sometimes purely cosmetic correction of metabolic acidosis. The metabolic acidosis of chronic renal failure is well tolerated and usually requires no treatment. In contrast, the hyperchloraemic acidosis of renal tubular acidosis should be carefully corrected by the long-term administration of base by mouth* in order to prevent hypokalaemia, rickets or osteomalacia, nephrocalcinosis and urolithiasis.

Diabetic ketoacidosis is corrected primarily by administering insulin and only in severe acidaemia (pH < 7.0) by giving sodium bicarbonate. Starvation ketosis and metabolic acidosis due to transient gastrointestinal problems or due to the administration of acetazolamide does not generally require correction.

Major lactic acidosis requires determined treatment of the causative disorder. Measures to improve tissue perfusion and the elimination of potentially causative drugs are of utmost importance. Whenever serum lactate exceeds 5 mmol/l, potentially enormous amounts of bicarbonate are required if plasma bicarbonate is to be kept above 10 mmol/l. Ancillary therapeutic measures include the administration of thiamine (thiamine deficiency, which is likely to occur in alcoholics, may limit pyruvate oxidation thereby contributing to LA) and insulin and glucose (2–3 units/h + glucose as needed) may decrease the plasma pyruvate concentration by increasing pyruvate oxidation and suppressing pyruvate formation.

Metabolic Alkalosis

In addition to excluding alkalinising medicines and attempting to correct the underlying problems, one of the most efficient measures (at least in the chloride-responsive variety of metabolic acidosis) is the administration of chloride, either as NaCl or KCl

---

* Shohl's solution (90 g crystalline sodium citrate, 140 g citric acid, water added to 1 l) containing the equivalent of 1 mmol NaHCO$_3$ per ml solution was long the customary treatment. Sodium bicarbonate or both sodium and potassium bicarbonate may be more convenient.

or both according to circumstances. Metabolic alkalosis due to primary mineralocorticoid excess is not corrected by providing chloride. In rare cases of severe metabolic alkalosis and on even rarer occasions of metabolic alkalosis with ECF excess, the use of hydrochloric acid (N/10 or N/20), administered via a central venous catheter, is justified. The rate of administration is determined by the extent of the hydrogen ion deficit. It should be carefully controlled and generally should not exceed 100 ml of N/10 HCl (corresponding to 10 mmol of H^+) per h. Arginine-HCl and lysine-HCl as a means of providing hydrogen ions offer no advantage over sodium chloride or, in extreme situations, hydrochloric acid. Because of the inherent danger of inducing acute hyperkalaemia they should be avoided.

C.

Therapeutic Measures

INTRAGASTRIC FEEDING

The feeding solution must be hypotonic or isotonic to body fluids. If it is hypertonic, water is drawn into the gut and has a bulk-purgative effect. In the absence of abnormal losses it is convenient to give about 50–60 mmol of sodium and potassium daily.

The diet must supply sufficient energy to enable nitrogen balance to be maintained. It is fruitless to increase protein intake without supplying sufficient energy for its utilisation. To supply 12 600 kJ (3000 kCal) with glucose alone would require 750 g of glucose, which, as a solution containing 50 g/l is isotonic, would require about 15 l of water to provide an isotonic feed, clearly an unrealistic proposition for intragastric feeding.

Fats and higher molecular weight carbohydrate sources (such as 'Caloreen', a mixture of glucose polymers which has only one-fifth of the osmolality of glucose in solution) are practical alternatives. Proteins, being of large molecular weight, make little contribution to the osmolality of the feed unlike aminoacids and peptides.

The water content of a tube feed is governed by the need to avoid a hypertonic solution, to replace insensible and abnormal losses and to provide for the excretion of the osmotic load presented to the kidney (*see* p. 19).

It is impracticable to give more than 3 l of tube feed daily. The composition of some readily available tube feeds is given in Table C.1.

Further Reading

Masterton J.P., Dudley H.A.F., Mac Rae S. (1963). Design of tube feeds for surgical patients. *Brit. Med. J.*; 2:909–13.

Table C.1

THE COMPOSITION OF READILY AVAILABLE TUBE-FEEDS

	Clinifeed 400 (vanilla) 5 cans	Vivonex standard 7 packets	Nutraxil 4 bottles	Isocal 6 cans
Carbohydrate (g)	275	483	276	283
Fat	67	3	68	94
Protein	75	44	76	72
Nitrogen	12	7	12	11
Energy (kcal)	2000	2100	2000	2130
(MJ)	8.4	9.1	8.4	9.1
Sodium	52	78	66	48
Potassium	61	63	64	72
Osmolarity (mmol/l)	306	550	300	300
Volume at full strength* (ml)	2500	2100	2000	2130

* It is usual to start with one-quarter strength and to build up both the quantity of feed and the concentration over a few days or weeks; quantity and concentration should not be increased simultaneously.

TOTAL PARENTERAL NUTRITION

Whenever the oral energy intake is insufficient to meet the patient's needs for longer than a few days the diet should be supplemented, if necessary by parenteral feeding. *Total* parenteral nutrition provides not only the total calorific requirements but simultaneously supplies all the necessary amino acids, vitamins, trace metals, haematinics, water and electrolytes. Patients should be carefully selected and the doctor in charge should not only be experienced but willing to commit himself to the patient and the task.

The Indications

Total parenteral nutrition (TPN) is considered when adequate intake is *impossible* (e.g. chronic alimentary tract obstruction, prolonged adynamic ileus, high output fistula after extensive bowel surgery, acute pancreatitis, massive resection of small bowel, major burns and other causes of massive catabolism etc.); when adequate enteral intake is *inadvisable* (e.g. exacerbation of inflammatory bowel disease, toxic megacolon, internal and external intestinal fistulae); when adequate enteral intake is *improbable* (e.g. anorexia nervosa, chronic starvation and severe mental depression) and when adequate enteral intake is *hazardous* (e.g. disorders of consciousness with regurgitation and tracheoesophageal fistulae).

Total parenteral nutrition is required by only a small minority of patients.

Requirements

The basic energy requirement of normal man amounts to 0.10–0.13 MJ/kg (25–30 kcal/kg) body weight. After massive trauma and major surgery the requirements approach 0.21 MJ/kg (50 kcal/kg). Accordingly the following average needs have been calculated: 8.4–12.6 MJ (2000–3000 kcal) after uncomplicated major surgery; 12.6–18.9 MJ (3000–4500 kcal) after severe trauma or after surgery complicated by sepsis; 14.5–>21 MJ (3500–>5000 kcal) after major burns. Meeting these energy requirements is the first goal of TPN because if caloric intake is inadequate the nitrogen balance will remain negative no matter how much protein or amino acids are supplied. As a general rule a minimum of 150 kcal should be given for every g of nitrogen infused.

The minimum daily nitrogen requirement of 3.5 g corresponds to 21 g of protein (1 g N = 6.25 g of protein). These requirements rapidly increase with trauma, surgery and infection, reaching 12–20 g of nitrogen after uncomplicated major surgery, 20–32 g of nitrogen after severe trauma or major surgery complicated by infection and sepsis, and >32 g of nitrogen in patients with major burns. Note that these amounts of nitrogen assume that all the total parenteral supply will be used for protein synthesis, a degree of efficiency which will not be reached.

The daily requirements for Mg^{++} (200–500 mg or 8–20 mmol), Ca^{++} (200–400 mg or 5–10 mmol), phosphate (200–400 mg or 6.5–13 mmol) are often supplied with the commercial amino acid solutions but may have to be added as $MgSO_4$ (50%, 2 mmol Mg^{++}/ml), Calcium gluconate (10%, 0.25 mmol Ca^{++}/ml), K_2HPO_4 (2 mmol K^+, 1 mmol HPO_4^{--} per ml).

The daily potassium requirements are variable and depend on the rate of glucose assimilation, urinary potassium losses and abnormal extrarenal potassium losses. In the absence of abnormal losses a daily supply of 4 mmol K^+/100 kcal (80–120 mmol K^+), given as K_2HPO_4 or KCl will meet the needs of most patients.

The requirements for salt and water in TPN are determined by the clinical situation. Since an adequate supply of calories and amino acids requires the infusion of at least 2500 ml of fluid (Table C.2) TPN may be limited by renal insufficiency.

Vitamin and trace metal requirements are covered by standard polyvitamin preparations. In addition, with prolonged TPN, the requirements for vitamin K_1 amount to 5–10 mg per week, B_{12} 100 μg/week and folic acid 3–6 mg/day, all three given i.m.

The Feeding Components

Carbohydrates

Glucose is the carbohydrate of choice; up to 1000 g are assimilated per day. As a general rule the infusion rate should not exceed 0.5 g/kg body weight per hour. If glucose tolerance is diminished (blood glucose >16 mmol/l during glucose infusion at a rate required for adequate TPN) or if blood glucose exceeds 9 mmol/l before starting TPN, insulin should be added to the infusion ('Actrapid' or an equivalent insulin, 1 u/4 g glucose). Depending on the response of the patient the dosage of insulin may be increased stepwise until blood glucose remains within the range of 5–10 mmol/l. The glucose load should be evenly infused throughout each 24 h period. A continuous infusion is mandatory whenever the addition of insulin is required. If the infusion is discontinued for any reason blood glucose should be monitored to detect and prevent serious hypoglycaemia.

While glucose has both biological and economical advantages, the difficulties of preparing sterile mixtures with amino acids have led to an intensive search for alternative carbohydrates.

Table C.2
THE COMPOSITION (PER LITRE) OF SOME SOLUTIONS COMMONLY USED FOR INTRAVENOUS NUTRITION

	Aminofusin			Aminoplex		Vamin			Synthamin				Trophysan	Intralipid	
	L600	L1000	Lforte	5	14	N	F	G	7S	9	14	17	L10	10%	20%
Aminoacids (g)	50	50	100	33	87	70	70	70	40	55	85	100	40		
Carbohydrate (g)															
Sorbitol	100	100		125					150						
Ethanol	50	50		50											
Fructose							100								
Glucose								100							
Fats (g)														100	200
Glycerol (g)														25	25
Electrolytes (mmol)															
Sodium	40	40	40	35	35	50	50	50	38	73	73	73	6		
Potassium	30	30	30	15	30	20	20	20	30	60	60	60	8		
Magnesium	5	5	5			1.5	1.5	1.5	2.5	5	5	5			
Calcium						2.5	2.5	2.5							
Acetate	10	10	10			55	55	55	60	100	130	150			
Malate	15	15	5												
Chloride	14	14	27	62	81	55	55	55	35	70	70	70	27		
Phosphate									15	30	30	30			
Nitrogen (g)	7.6	7.6	15.2	5	13.4	9.4	9.4	9.4	6.7	9.3	14.3	16.9	6.7		
Energy															
(kcal)	600	1000	400	1000	340	250	650	650	760	220	320	400	570	1100	2000
(kJ)	2500	4200	1700	4200	1400	1047	2700	2700	3181	916	1330	1660	2370	4600	8400
Osmolality (mmol/kg)	1300	1500	1020	2415	875	700	1260	1260	1150	850	1160	1300	1000	280	330
pH	6.8	6.8	5.4	7.4	7.4	5.2	5.2	5.2	6.0	6.0	6.0	6.0	6.2–6.7		

Fructose, sorbitol, xylitol and ethanol have all been used but their disadvantages outweigh their advantages.

Fat emulsions

These have made it possible to administer large amounts of calories without fluid overload: 500 ml of a 20% fat emulsion (mainly soy-bean preparations) provide approximately 4.2 MJ (1000 kcal). Fat emulsions also supply the small quantities of essential fatty acids needed. The osmolality of fat emulsions is low and due only to a small amount of carbohydrate or glycerin contained in commercial solutions. Since fat tolerance may be limited initially, fat emulsions are preferably not added until at least 24 h after initiation of parenteral nutrition. Even then the daily amount of fat administered should be slowly increased, starting with 0.5 g/kg body weight, aiming at a total of 2 g/kg per day. In order to secure optimum fat assimilation, the infusion should be spread over a number of hours (total daily amount within not less than 5 h). In the event of lipid intolerance shown by lipaemia persisting 12 h after completing infusion, the duration of the infusion should be prolonged, the daily dose reduced, and/or a break should be allowed to complete clearing of lipaemia. Side effects include nausea, pyrogenic reactions, flushing, urticaria and headache, hyperlipidaemia, liver damage, anaemia, coagulation disorders and diminished bacterial defence. Accordingly, severe diffuse liver damage, hyperlipidaemia and pregnancy are considered contraindications against the use of fat emulsions. In addition it is advisable not to use fats in patients with manifest haemorrhagic diathesis.

Protein/amino acids

Hydrolysates of biological proteins such as casein, have largely been replaced by mixtures of synthetic crystalline l-amino acids. It does not seem to matter whether the pattern of amino acid composition follows that of plasma or the minimum requirements for each amino acid calculated by Rose.

1 g of amino acids per kg body weight is generally adequate for a postoperative patient.

Commercial amino acid preparations contain different

amounts of electrolytes (*see* Table C.2). Their pH is usually low and their titratable acidity high. Thus they may cause metabolic acidosis, particularly when renal function is poor.

The Technique

Since most solutions used in total parenteral nutrition are markedly hyperosmolar and/or acidic (*see* Table C.2) they must be administered through a central venous catheter to avoid thrombophlebitis. A peripheral line may suffice for supplemental parenteral feeding and for fat solutions, which are approximately isotonic. Positioning the catheter, daily catheter care and the handling of the lines and bottles requires stringent aseptic techniques. The catheter should be changed whenever there is inflammation at the site of insertion, signs of local thrombophlebitis or significant fever for which no other cause can be found. The catheter tip should always be cultured after removal. 1 ml of heparin sodium (1000 u) added to each bottle of hypertonic glucose may inhibit local venous thrombosis, prolong catheter life and enhance clearing of the lipids.

The Programme

The daily caloric and nitrogen requirement is given evenly throughout a full 24 h period. Electrolyte and water needs not covered by the carbohydrate, fat and amino acid solutions are given as additives to the carbohydrate bottles or as an additional fluid volume of appropriate composition.

Start parenteral nutrition with a low caloric load, e.g. 4.2 MJ/day (1000 kcal/day), then gradually increase to the required total intake. With glucose intolerance during the early phase of parenteral nutrition reduce the carbohydrate load by 50% and increase again stepwise and under close control of blood glucose concentrations (*see* p. 156). Add water-soluble vitamins, fat-soluble vitamins, and trace elements daily. Add fat emulsions 24–48 h after commencing parenteral nutrition and not before. Do not use amino acid solutions without providing an adequate caloric intake.

Table C.3
VARIOUS REGIMENS OF TPN

Bottles							Contents/500 ml bottle	MJ	Volume infused (ml)	Carbo-hydrate (g)	Nitro-gen (g)	Fat (g)	Elements (mmol) Na	K	Cl	Mg	Ca	Zn	Mn	PO_4
2							Synthamin 14	0.74		–	7.15	–	37	30	35	2.5	–	–	–	15
1	2	1	1		1	2	Vamin glucose*	1.36		50	4.7		25	10	28	0.8	1.3			
		1	1	2	1		Aminosol 10%*	0.69			6.4		63	0.2	60			0.01		9
1	1	1	1	1	1	1	Electrolyte solution A with 20% w/v dextrose†	1.67		100					27	14	13	0.04	0.02	
	1	1	1	1	1	1	Electrolyte solution B with 20% w/v dextrose†	1.67		100				30						30
1.5	1	1	1				Dextrose 50%	4.18		250										
1	1	1		1	1	1	Intralipid 20%*	4.18				100								
							Low sodium	10.24	2500	300	9.4	100	50	50	83	15.5	16	0.04	0.02	30
							Standard	9.57	2500	250	11.1	100	93	40	115	14.8	14	0.05	0.02	39
							High sodium	8.90	2500	200	12.8	100	136	30	147	14	13	0.06	0.02	48
							Fat-free	9.57	2500	500	11.1		93	40	115	14.8	14	0.05	0.02	39
							Increased calories	13.75	3000	500	11.1	100	93	40	115	14.8	14	0.05	0.02	39
							Increased caloires, low Na	14.42	3000	550	9.4	100	50	50	83	15.5	16	0.04	0.02	30
							Increased calories high protein	14.12	3250	475	19.0	100	98	70	98	19.8	14.3	0.01	0.02	30

* KabiVitrum Ltd † Travenol Ltd Conversion: SI to traditional units – Energy: 1 MJ = 238 kcal

Notes: 1. The top of the Table shows the content of the bottles used. Below is an analysis of the different regimens that can be formulated.

2. If a patient's sodium loss is unknown, especially if they have recently undergone surgery, start on the 'low sodium' regimen. When there is evidence of sodium loss of more than 80 or 120 mmol/24 h then the 'standard' or 'high sodium' regimens may be used, respectively. Note that these also contain a greater amount of nitrogen.

3. Should the increased calorie high protein regimen be used, electrolytes (Na, K, Mg, PO_4), acid base status and blood glucose must be monitored most carefully. Insulin is invariably required to maintain a blood glucose between 8.0 and 10.0 mmol/l.

4. The fat emulsion should be started after the daily blood samples have been taken and should also finish during the day so that the nursing staff can change the drip set and dressing during daylight hours.

5. Additives must not be put in the fat emulsion. Check all additives for compatibility. If in doubt contact Pharmacy.

6. The phosphate content of the fat emulsion has been omitted since it is uncertain whether it is freely available.

(Modified from Ellis *et al.* 1976 by Hanson, 1979 reproduced by permission of Blackwell Scientific Publications.)

Table C.3 illustrates an approach to the selection and assembling of various commonly required regimens using commercially available solutions.

The Complications and Dangers
(Table C.4)

Table C.4
COMPLICATIONS DURING PARENTERAL NUTRITION

Catheter sepsis and septic venous thrombosis
Severe hyperosmolality
Hypokalaemia
Hypophosphataemia
Hypomagnesaemia
Folic acid deficiency
Essential fatty acid deficiency

Infection and septicaemia are the major threat and cannot be entirely eliminated. In addition to bacterial infections systemic mycoses should also be considered. Febrile reactions are frequent and do not necessarily indicate infection.

Hyperosmolality is a constant risk and is mainly due to severe hyperglycaemia. A rapid increase in total osmolality above 360 mmol/kg (corresponding to a hyperglycaemia of 60 mmol/l in the presence of normal plasma electrolytes) is potentially lethal and blood glucose should not be allowed to rise above 25 mmol/l. A rising serum sodium may contribute to the hyperosmolality. More often it is a consequence of water deficit from osmotic diuresis rather than the result of sodium excess.

Hypokalaemia, hypomagnesaemia and phosphorus deficiency

These mainly result from an increased requirement during tissue anabolism. Folic acid depletion should be suspected if there is leukopenia and/or thrombocytopenia, particularly in alcoholic patients, patients on folate antagonists or patients undergoing dialysis. Essential fatty acid deficiency occasionally occurs during prolonged fat-free parenteral nutrition. The predominant skin lesions, a scaly dermatitis, are prevented or treated by local application of sunflower seed oil, when fat emulsions are contraindicated.

The *monitoring of laboratory data* is particularly important when rapid changes are apt to occur, i.e. during the initiation of the feeding programme and with intercurrent changes of the clinical condition.

1. *Glucose.* During the initial phase the urine should be tested for glucose frequently (every 6 h). Blood sugar is measured whenever the urine sugar exceeds 1% – initially at least once a day; in a more stable situation once or twice a week.

2. *Electrolytes.* Serum electrolytes should be checked every other day after the initial phase of treatment and whenever the clinical condition of the patient changes.

3. *Serum creatinine* and *blood urea* are measured twice a week or whenever acute changes occur. During the initial phase daily measurements are recommended.

4. *Acid-base measurements* are undertaken daily during the early phase of TPN, particularly with borderline renal function and when high nitrogen regimens are used. Later these variables are checked once a week.

5. The *full blood count, haemoglobin and platelets* should be measured daily during the initiation of TPN and later twice a week.

6. *Liver function tests* are obtained twice a week during the initial phase and once weekly thereafter.

7. Calcium, phosphorus, osmolality, blood cultures and body weight are measured twice weekly initially then weekly.

Further Reading

Dudrick S.J., Long J.M. (1977). Applications and hazards of intravenous hyperalimentation. *Ann. Rev. Med*; **28**:517–28.

Dudrick S.J., Wilmore D.W., Vars H.M. *et al.* (1968). Long-term total parenteral nutrition with growth and development and positive nitrogen balance. *Surgery*; **64**:134–42.

Ellis B.W., Stanbridge R.L., Fielding L.P., Dudley H.A.F. (1976). A rational approach to parenteral nutrition. *Brit. Med. J*; **1**:1388–91.

Göschke H., Grötzinger U., Nosbaum J.A., Leutenegger A., Gigon J. P. (1973). Belastbarkeit des Glucosestoffwechsels bei intravenöser Hyperalimentation. *Schweiz Med Wschr*; **103**:1228–34.

Hanson G. C. (1979). Intravenous nutrition – indications and management. In *Clinical Medicine and Therapeutics II* (Richards P., Mather H., eds.) pp. 203–14. Oxford: Blackwell Scientific.
Lee H.A. (1974). *Parenteral Nutrition in Acute Metabolic Illness*. London: Academic Press.

PERITONEAL DIALYSIS

The only satisfactory way to learn the technique of peritoneal dialysis is to perform it under experienced supervision. The purpose of this section is only to outline the principles involved.

The aim is to remove excess ECF from a patient with acute or chronic renal failure, to treat hyperkalaemia and/or to eliminate toxic products of protein metabolism responsible for the syndrome of uraemia. It is also occasionally used to eliminate poisons.

At its simplest, the technique involves the insertion of a teflon catheter under local anaesthetic into the peritoneal cavity; a site in the midline 2 cm below the umbilicus is the most usual. The catheter tip is directed deep into the pelvis. One or two litres of dialysate are run in by gravity, retained for a variable dwell time and siphoned off again. Glucose is used to make the dialysate hypertonic and, therefore, to extract extracellular fluid. Three glucose strengths are generally available (*see* Table C.5).

Most of the movements of salt and water take place in the first 20 min which is a suitable dwell time if the prime object of dialysis is gently to remove salt and water. But a greater volume can be extracted if drainage begins as soon as the dialysate has been delivered into the peritoneal cavity and each cycle is restricted to 1 h or less. The maximum diffusion of urea and other small molecules is also rapid but substantial diffusion continues for at least 30 min which is a suitable dwell time when relief of uraemia is the prime object.

Initially total cycle times of 1.5 h are convenient: a rapid run-in, a dwell time of 20 to 30 min, and the remainder of the period to allow full siphonage. Later, when fluid balance is satisfactory and maintenance of control of uraemia is all that is desired the total cycle time can well be lengthened to 2 h, of which 40–60 min is dwell time. A more rapid fluid shift is

Table C.5
PERITONEAL DIALYSIS SOLUTIONS

	Diaflex 61	*Diaflex 62*	*Diaflex 63* *(low sodium)*
Dextrose BP (g/l)	13.6	63.6	13.6
Sodium (mmol/l)	141	142	131
Calcium (mmol/l)	1.8	1.8	1.8
Magnesium (mmol/l)	0.75	0.75	0.75
Chloride (mmol/l)	100	100	100
Lactate (mmol/l)	45	45	45
Osmolality (mmol/kg)	365	643	343

	Dianeal with Dextrose 1.36%	*Dianeal with Dextrose 3.86%*
Dextrose BP (g/l)	13.6	38.6
Sodium (mmol/l)	140	140
Calcium (mmol/l)	1.8	1.8
Magnesium (mmol/l)	0.7	0.7
Chloride (mmol/l)	101	101
Lactate (mmol/l)	45	45
Osmolality (mmol/kg)	364	504

achieved with the 6.36 g/dl glucose solution, but it is sufficiently hypertonic to cause discomfort and is best avoided; under these circumstances the use of a solution containing 3.86 g/dl makes a comfortable and satisfactory compromise. For normal maintenance 6 or 8 two-litre exchanges daily are usually sufficient.

Peritoneal dialysis removes fluid by 'bulk flow' of water and solutes, the solutes moving more slowly than water. The faster the fluid transfer the more hypotonic the fluid transferred and therefore the greater the risk of the patient becoming hypernatraemic. Thus, peritoneal dialysis extracts saline at slightly lower than plasma concentration. If too much fluid is extracted it must be replaced by normal saline or by 5% dextrose if the patient becomes hypernatraemic.

Glucose moves continuously in the opposite direction along the concentration gradient. Indeed so substantial is the glucose absorption that patients sometimes develop sufficiently severe hyperglycaemia to become confused from intracellular dehydration.

Inadvertently peritoneal dialysis can cause fluid overload because of poor drainage and when hyponatraemic patients are dialysed with a dialysate containing 140 mmol Na$^+$/l. Sodium passes from dialysate to ECF although the hypertonicity of the dialysate prevents water from moving with it. The increase in ECF sodium results in an internal transfusion of water from ICF to ECF which may expand plasma volume sufficiently to cause heart failure. Thus hyponatraemic patients should be dialysed initially against dialysate with a lower sodium concentration; a suitable solution is available, in which the sodium concentration is 131 mmol/l.

Potassium chloride should be added to peritoneal dialysis solutions in a concentration not greater than 5 mmol/l when the plasma potassium falls below 4 mmol/l. A rapid reduction in plasma potassium should be avoided in digitalised patients.

Further Reading

Colombi A. (1980). *Die Peritonealdialyse*. Stuttgart: Enke.

Maher J.F. (1980). Peritoneal transport rates: mechanisms, limitations and methods for augmentation. *Kidney Int*; 18(suppl. 10):S117–20.

Nolph K.D., Miller F., Rubin J., Popovich R. (1980). New directions in peritoneal dialysis concepts and applications. *Kidney Int*; 18 (suppl. 10):S111–6.

Nolph K.D., Popovich R.P., Moncrief J.W. (1978). Theoretical and practical implications of continuous ambulatory peritoneal dialysis. *Nephron*; 21:117–23.

Nolph K.D., Twardowski Z.J., Popovich R.P., Rubin. (1979). Equilibration of peritoneal dialysis solutions during long dwell exchanges. *J. Lab. Clin. Med*; 93:246–57.

Oreopoulos D.G., Robson M., Faller B., Ogilvie R., Rapaport A., de Veber G.A. (1979). Continuous ambulatory peritoneal dialysis: a new era in the treatment of chronic renal failure. *Clin. Nephrol*; 11:125–9.

Popovich R.P., Moncrief J.W., Nolph K.D., Ghods A.J., Twardowski Z.J., Pyle W.K. (1978). Continuous ambulatory peritoneal dialysis. *Ann. Intern. Med*; 88:449–56.

FORCED ALKALINE DIURESIS

Forced alkaline diuresis is effective treatment for severe salicylate and phenobarbitone poisoning. Both are weak acids and their elimination by non-ionic diffusion is increased by alkalinising tubular fluid. Care must be taken not to overload the circulation or to cause hypokalaemia. It is important, however, to make allowance for the fact that patients with severe salicylate overdosage are usually severely water and, to a lesser extent, sodium depleted as a result of hyperventilation, sweating and vomiting. Accurate hourly charting of fluid balance is essential. The bladder should be catheterised and central venous pressure measurement is desirable.

Recommended Procedure

1. Assure a clear airway and provide assisted ventilation if necessary.
2. Aspirate the stomach.
3. Give plasma, if the patient is poorly perfused and oliguric. Do not give vasoconstrictors.
4. Determine plasma urea (plasma creatinine) and electrolytes in all cases. Perform arterial blood gas analysis in patients with salicylate poisoning (the alkaline diuresis may need to be modified according to the results).
5. Subject to a normal plasma sodium concentration give 500 ml 1 N (1.4%) sodium bicarbonate and 500 ml 5% dextrose on half-hourly rotation until the plasma salicylate concentration is less than 50 mg/100 ml or a patient with phenobarbitone overdose has recovered consciousness. Give elderly patients 20 mg of frusemide i.v. at the outset. Check urine pH periodically to ensure that it is above 7.5.
6. Replace potassium chloride at rate of 13–27 mmol (1–2 g)/h. Check plasma potassium at 2 h and later if necessary.
7. Give frusemide 20 mg i.v. whenever input exceeds output by 1.5 l or if signs of pulmonary congestion or heart failure develop*. If positive balance reaches 2 l reduce the rate of infusion.
8. Frequent clinical examination of the chest ensures early diagnosis of pulmonary congestion.

* An alternative is to give mannitol 10% or 20% solution over 10–20 min ... probably sa...

* An alternative is to give mannitol 10% or 20% at an infusion rate sufficient to produce a urinary flow rate of about 4ml per minute when diuresis slows but the use of a diuretic is simpler and safer.

Index

167